GW00322177

Women's Health Guide

Ann Furedi

Mary Tidyman

This book is dedicated to women everywhere, and in particular to Ann's mum, Joan, and to Mary's daughters, Annie and Polly, as they reach the threshold of womanhood.

Copyright © 1994 Ann Furedi and Mary Tidyman

British Library Cataloguing in Publication Data
Furedi, Ann
Women's Health Guide
I. Title II. Tidyman, Mary III. Mills, Siri
613.0424

ISBN 1 85448 933 X (paperback)
ISBN 1 85448 992 5 (hardback)

The right of Ann Furedi and Mary Tidyman to be identified as the authors of this work has been asserted by them in accordance with the Copyright, Designs and Patents Act 1988.

All rights reserved. No part of this publication may be reproduced in any material form (including photocopying or storing it in any medium by electronic means and whether or not transiently or incidently to some other use of this publication) without the prior written permission of the copyright owners, except in accordance with the provisions of the Copyright, Designs and Patents Act 1998 or under the terms of a licence issued by the Copyright Licensing Agency, 90 Tottenham Court Road, London W1P 9HE. Applications for the copyright owners' written permission to reproduce any part of this publication should be addressed in the first instance to the publisher.

The views expressed in this publication are those of the authors and are not necessarily those of the Health Education Authority.

Designed by
John and Orna Designs
Principal photography by
Caroline Mardon
Illustrations by Siri Mills
First published 1994
Typeset by
Wordbase Ltd, London
Printed in England for
Health Education Authority
Hamilton House
Mabledon Place
London WC1H 9TX

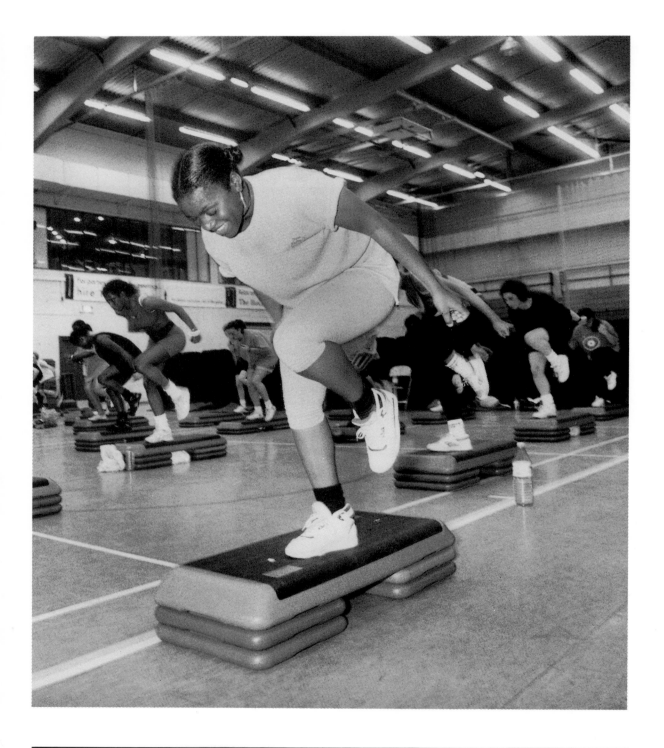

Good health is not something that can be separated from the rest of our lives. A multitude of different factors contributes to our well-being and, by understanding their influence, we can try to take control of our health.

All the following have a major influence on our health and well-being.

Lifestyle •

We know that our lifestyle is intimately bound up with our general health. Study after study shows that exercise is good for our heart, our lungs and our circulation in addition to toning and strengthening our muscles. We are bombarded with advice about healthy eating and constantly reminded to give up smoking and cut down drinking.

Sometimes the gap between how we *should* live and how we do live seems too wide to bridge. It seems easier simply to carry on and to go on hoping for the best than to make even some of the changes we know would be good for us.

A healthier lifestyle requires calculations and compromises. We all know someone who, every January, makes the same New Year's resolutions: to give up smoking and drinking, to cut down on caffeine, to swim three times a week, and to change to skimmed milk. By February the good intentions have either been forgotten or deliberately abandoned on the grounds that 'it's all too much'. It is far better to weigh up which changes you think you can make to enhance your life, and succeed, than to overhaul everything and flunk out. To calculate which are the *essential* changes and to work out where you can compromise you need to understand what benefits you are likely to achieve. The more we know about the way our bodies respond to the way we live, the more we can work out a healthy programme for living.

Work •

Work away from the home plays a major part in the lives of more and more women. Most women today juggle their lives between a job and a family and the strain can take its toll.

A job can make a positive contribution to our well-being if it increases our confidence and sense of self-worth. A decent wage can enhance our lifestyle by making it easier for us to make ends meet or, if we are lucky, allowing us to indulge in new leisure pursuits and take relaxing holidays.

But work can also damage our health. For example, office technologies create new potential problems such as repetitive strain injury. If you understand how your job can affect your health you can take steps to compensate for it. For example, if technology has made your job more sedentary you may feel you want to make a special effort to exercise. Knowledge about how your job can affect your health gives you the ability to discuss with your employer or your union how any potential risks can be minimised.

Relationships •

Our relationships with friends, lovers, children, relatives and colleagues have an enormous effect on our well-being. Human beings are social animals. We have an urge to share our thoughts and feelings with others and to participate in their joys and sorrows in return. Our relationships with other people help to shape our view of ourselves, and our attitude to ourselves can make the difference between feeling on the top of the world or at the bottom.

Our relationships can enable or disable us. They can be positive influences by giving us confidence to strike out and make our own way, or they can be negative by making us feel bad about ourselves. How we feel others view us can have a perceptible effect on our well-being. If we feel we are loved and have the support and respect of others it is easier to take control when health problems occur. If we feel we are worthless and isolated, a minor infection can seem too much to bear.

Sometimes if we understand the dynamic between our self-esteem and our well-being we can shake ourselves out of the doldrums and refuse to submit to negative feelings.

Age •   We often worry that as we grow older our health will fail and, of course, it might. But old age and ill health are not necessarily bedfellows. Greater understanding of the changes in our bodies during middle age helps us to make the most of our later life.

If you are reasonably healthy and fit, retirement can be a new beginning. if we know the possible problems we can prepare to meet them head on. For example, you can ease the problem of stiff joints if you get into the habit of regular gentle exercise. Developments in medical technology mean that we can defeat the problems that would have immobilised people just a generation ago.

Illness •   However careful we are to adopt a healthy way of life, illness can strike. Sometimes it's obvious that we are ill, but sometimes we dither and debate about whether there is anything wrong at all. If you are stricken with flu your temperature soars, you feel achy and shivery and as you crawl into bed you know that there is a problem. But when you have a small lump in your breast, or an irritating vaginal discharge, or period pains that are more severe than normal, it is often hard to decide whether to seek medical advice or just to wait and see.

It is easier to resolve these dilemmas if we understand a little about how our body works. For example, if you understand the effects of your hormones on your breasts throughout your monthly cycle you are less likely to be worried by the 'normal' swelling and tenderness that many of us suffer before our period. Knowing what the symptoms of endometriosis are, you are more likely to seek help and to discover what treatments are on offer.

Taking Control

All the above factors mould our well-being. We can make a special effort to take control of our health to counter the negative influences and enhance the good ones.

Of course there are lots of things that it is not possible to control. Poverty is probably one of the greatest influences on health today. If low income means that you live in a damp house which you can ill afford to heat, then it may be impossible to avoid certain health problems. But many of us can enhance our health if we take the trouble to find out how to do it.

This book looks at the main influences that affect our health. It is not a comprehensive medical encyclopaedia, nor does it provide a top to toe study of how your body works. The *Women's Health Guide* provides you with the basic information you need as a first step to finding out more. It may not provide you with all the answers, but it will provide you with the information you need to obtain further knowledge. Often we don't get the answers we need from doctors because we don't know how to phrase the questions. We miss out on advice and support because we don't know where to obtain it. The information this book provides will enable you to find out more.

There are many issues of relevance to women's health that are not covered in these pages. For example, there is nothing on having a baby or rearing children, two issues which dominate the lives of most women. However, because they are significant to our lives, the bookshelves are loaded with volumes on precisely these issues and we felt the *Women's Health Guide* could more usefully look at issues on which less information was available.

As women we are often so busy caring for other people that we neglect our own health needs. It's time to take time for ourselves!

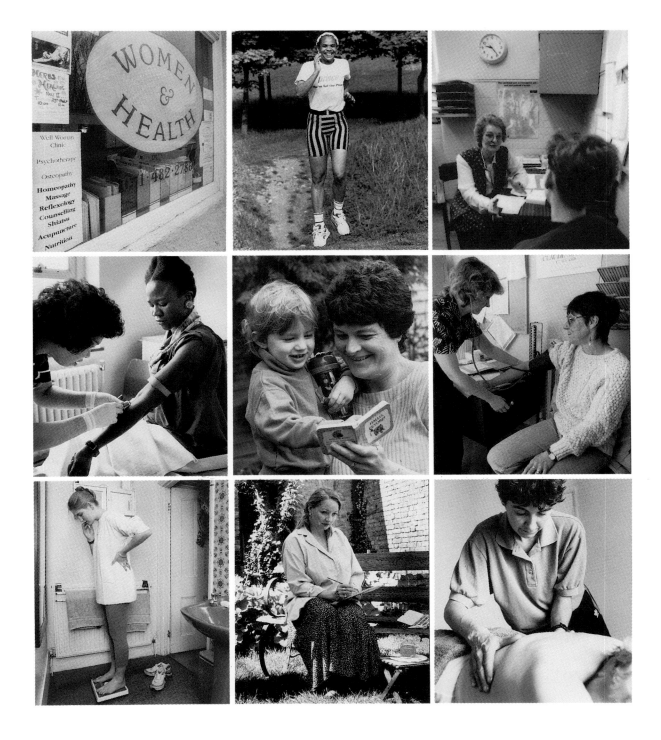

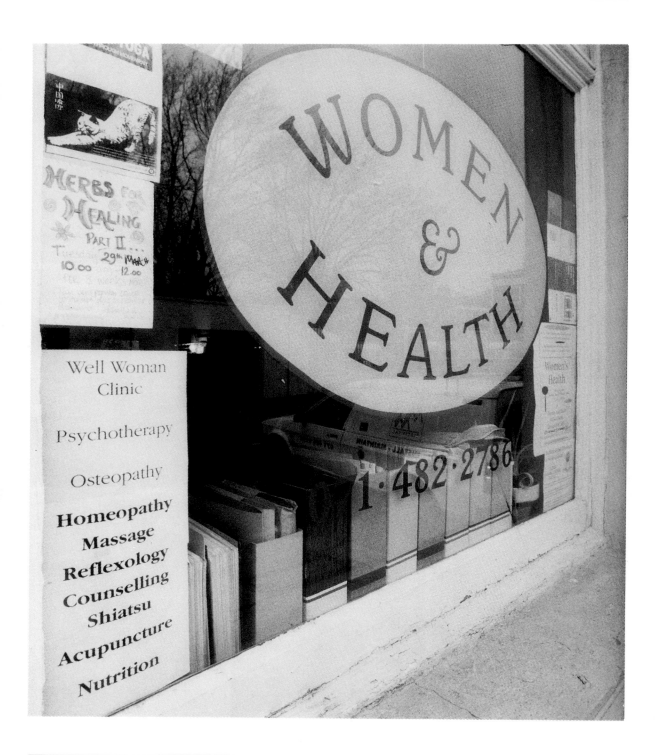

A Woman's Mental Health

Feeling well is not just tied up with physical health. It's also how you feel about yourself, your relationships with others, and your ability to cope with the inevitable stresses and problems which life throws at you. Your body and mind are tuned into each other, so that being physically unwell can easily cause you to feel anxious or depressed. Similarly, stress may contribute to a variety of physical health problems.

Mental health problems are a major cause of illness, distress and disability, making significant demands on health and social services. They account for around 14 per cent of NHS inpatient costs. About 50 per cent of social workers' caseloads involve people with a mental health problem. Mental health problems also account for about 80 million days' sick leave each year, leading to significant costs to employers, and to society as a whole.

Women tend to suffer more than men from certain types of mental health problems, in particular from depression and anxiety. Around twice as many women as men use mental health services, and 58 per cent of people admitted as inpatients are women. One possible explanation for this is that women are more in touch with their feelings and more ready to seek help for their problems. Because we use the health service more than men anyway, for ourselves, our children and others we care for, we perhaps find it easier to turn to doctors for help with mental health problems. But it's likely that, as well as seeking help more readily, we actually do have poorer mental health than men, and this may well be because of the stresses and difficulties which we have to cope with, compounded by a general lack of power and choice in our lives.

Mental health problems are more common amongst socially disadvantaged groups, being particularly prevalent in areas of poor housing, overcrowding and few amenities. Certain black and minority ethnic groups have high rates of mental health problems, which may be explained in part by economic deprivation, and the racism and discrimination to which we are subjected. There is also concern that lack of cultural understanding and racial stereotyping actually leads to different responses and treatment for black people. For example, African-Caribbeans in the UK are more likely to be admitted to a psychiatric hospital, and are diagnosed as schizophrenic between three to six times more often than the white population, while the same scale of problem does not exist in Jamaica.

The suicide rate amongst women is half that of men. If you are a mother with young children then, statistically, you are likely to suffer from depression, but unlikely to commit suicide. However, more women than men kill themselves as they grow older. Around 90 per cent of people committing suicide have some kind of mental health disorder. The ending of marriages or partnerships – either by divorce or death – has a direct impact on suicide rates. Suicide is high in Asian women, with rates for those between 15 and 24 being more than double the national levels.

How You See Yourself

Self-esteem

We all have a basic need for love. Our feelings about ourselves stem from the love and care we receive as a child. Lack of affection during childhood can lead to problems in relationships and mental health when you grow up. Positive experiences which make you feel valued and wanted lead you to begin to develop a view of yourself as someone who is valuable and worthy of love, and your self-esteem grows.

The trouble is that if your self-esteem is poorly developed, or gets knocked, it's easy to believe that you are responsible for everything that goes wrong, making you wary of trying anything new, and giving you a pessimistic outlook on life. Low self-esteem can lead to passive or aggressive behaviour. When you feel low and lack confidence, it's harder to get your needs acknowledged. It's much more difficult to assert yourself, and you may find yourself putting up with things you don't like because you feel other people's feelings and needs are more important than your own.

Other people's expectations of how we should be and what we should do can affect the way we see ourselves. Low self-esteem may be linked to unrealistic expectations you have of yourself or which others impose on you – in your role as mother, partner, daughter, or employee. Remember, you don't have to prove anything and it's all right to make mistakes. Try to look for the good things rather than being over-critical of yourself.

Feeling positive about yourself can make you more likely to take on challenges, cope with problems and develop strong relationships where your needs as well as those of others are met. Take time to think through your strengths and abilities – the personal qualities you are most proud of, the things you do well, and the qualities which make your relationships positive. It's only when you begin to value yourself and put your own needs first that you can also give others the love and care which you choose to give them.

Expressing feelings

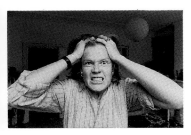

Women are not encouraged to express negative feelings such as anger, frustration and sadness. Instead, these feelings may be turned inwards, sometimes leading to stress and depression. You may feel guilty for the feelings you have, and try to hide them because they are not socially acceptable. There is an enormous amount of pressure on women to 'cope' and because some feelings may get in the way of this if expressed, it may seem better to bury them. But it's rather like a pressure cooker with too great a build-up of steam – there's danger of an explosion.

Sometimes, the events which trigger an explosion of anger are quite minor and entirely out of proportion to the amount of rage you feel. Your pent-up frustrations escape, leaving both you and the people around you bewildered. The trouble is that there's no way for other people to know how you feel about a particular situation if you don't express your true feelings at the time. Some women actually never allow their anger, frustration or sadness to show. They maintain a mask of controlled submissiveness rather than risk being judged uncaring by others. But bottling up your emotions in this way can leave you feeling stressed, anxious and depressed.

Once you find ways to express your feelings, depression may lift and you will feel much better. It may not always feel safe to show how you feel, but in the long run it's the only way you can be true to yourself. If it seems too difficult, share your feelings with friends, or find a sympathetic listener. You may need help to explore some of the feelings you have buried for so long. Professional counselling can help put you in touch with your feelings in an environment where it is safe to express them. You will begin to understand yourself more and become clearer about your own needs.

Relationships

Building good relationships

Positive mental health is often determined by the success or otherwise of our attempts to form and maintain relationships. As social beings, we all need other people to provide us with affection, and make us feel that we belong and are loved. The strength and quality will vary from one relationship to another. Most of us want and need to be close to someone, and one other person, perhaps, but not necessarily, a sexual partner, may be our main source of intimacy and emotional support. We may have a few close friends or family members in whom we can confide and share our joys and troubles. Beyond these special relationships may be a wider network of family and friends who offer social contact and friendship. Not all women have the intimate relationships and social support they need, and many feel isolated and lonely.

A positive and supportive relationship with a partner can be ideal for providing the intimacy which is so necessary for mental health. But research on married couples has shown that while married men have better mental health than single men, the reverse is true for women. There seems to be something about marriage, and presumably the same goes for any long-term relationship with a man and woman living together, which actually makes women more prone to stress, depression and other mental health problems. Women who have a difficult relationship with their partner, or who are on their own, may develop close, confiding relationships with friends or relatives, especially other women. They often find it helpful to talk to each other about marriage and relationship problems, children, health matters. Discovering that you are not the only one who slams doors or suffers from period problems can be very reassuring, and the intimacy which springs from this kind of exchange is also a good buffer against stress.

Improving the quality of your existing relationships or developing new ones may help you avoid or cope better with mental health problems. It's very easy to take relationships for granted, but they do need working at, however long-standing they are. It's important to feel positive about yourself in order to have the confidence to make the necessary changes. It may be a question of putting a bit more effort into existing relationships – paying more attention and finding more time to spend with the people you care about and do the things you enjoy together. Or you may want to make new friendships. One way of getting to know someone is to share information about yourself. Trusting somebody with personal information in this way tends to increase their trust in you, so that they also feel able to reveal personal things.

Feeling lonely

A study of women between the ages of 16 and 60 in 1978 found that one woman in four felt lonely, and if older women had been included in the sample this figure would probably have been higher still. Anyone can be lonely. You may be living in a house full of people, or on your own; your children may have left home, or you may be overstretched with family commitments; you may be separated or widowed, or you may live with someone you can't get close to; you may have a disability which prevents you from getting about and meeting people, or be tied to the house through caring for someone else; or you may be working in a poorly paid job with unsocial hours and no time or energy for a social life.

If you have young children and no paid work outside the home, you may have very little social contact with others. A good relationship with a partner can obviously provide a great deal of the emotional support and practical help which you need. Many fathers involve themselves in raising their children, and play an active part in caring for them and sharing general household tasks. Yet if they have a job, they may be out for much of the day, leaving you literally 'holding the baby'. Many men still see children and housework as 'women's work', leaving you to bear the brunt of it, whether or not you also have paid work. If you are one of the growing number of women who head a single-parent family (more than 90 per cent are headed by women), you may feel even more alone, especially if you are tired and struggling to make ends meet.

For women at home all day, it's easy to feel cut off from the adult world, spending many hours on your own or with only the children for company. If you have young children, getting out can be a major hassle, especially if you don't have the use of a car. Just getting ready to go out can be an exhausting exercise! And once out, shops and public transport are not well designed for prams or pushchairs, and many public places are not very welcoming towards children.

Developing a network of friends can be a particularly useful antidote to stress for women with young children, especially if you are coping on your own. The practical help and support you can offer each other in the way of babysitting, school runs, and other shared tasks helps relieve some of the physical strain, while being able to share problems and pool ideas can provide much-needed emotional support. It's not always easy to know where to start to make new friends, especially if you're lonely. Post-natal support groups, mother and toddler groups, and playgroups may all be good places to meet other women in a similar situation. There are a number of befriending schemes run by voluntary agencies to help lessen the isolation which many women feel – organisations such as the National Childbirth Trust, Homestart and Newpin may have groups in your area, and you can find out about them through your GP, health visitor, or in the local phone book.

Difficult relationships

Sometimes women find themselves locked into a relationship which offers little emotional sustenance or companionship, or at worst actually causes them a great deal of emotional distress. If your partner is manipulative, over-controlling, violent, or just cold and detached, you may need to think of ways to change the situation. If there are areas of a relationship that you are not happy with, then it will help to think about what your needs are and what you hope to get from the relationship. It is possible to make changes, but you need to be open about your needs and willing to communicate them clearly and honestly. It may feel safer to put up with the way things are, but that may only lead to frustration and discontent.

When trying to communicate about relationship problems, it helps to:

- Choose the right time
- Present any problems in a constructive way, and be specific and tactful
- Explain how the other person's behaviour is affecting you rather than assuming they know
- Anticipate their response, negotiate and reach compromises

It may seem too daunting to confront a difficult relationship on your own. It can help to share your problems and get some support from someone you can trust and confide in – a close friend or relative, or a counsellor. It may help to choose someone who has been through a similar situation, for instance, divorce, bereavement or breakdown, and who therefore understands what you are going through. Talking may help you to begin to understand some of your feelings and to think through what alternatives you may have. Strangely enough, support from family and friends may sometimes evaporate just when you need it most.

'My marriage had been going through difficulties for some time, but when I discovered John was having an affair it reached crisis point. Suddenly, I found my family and friends didn't want to know. I'm not sure if it was because they didn't know how to react, or were afraid to take sides, but I felt suddenly very isolated.'

If you are afraid of over-burdening your friends with your problems, or you don't have anyone you can talk to about very personal matters, then professional help is available. While friends can be a marvellous source of comfort and support, it sometimes needs professional help to get to the root of your problems and to identify positive ways forward. There may be a counselling service available at your GP's surgery or health centre, or your doctor may be able to help you find one.

Some voluntary agencies provide counselling. Relate, formerly known as the Marriage Guidance Council, is widely available across the UK and offers counselling to anyone with relationship problems. It helps if both you and your partner are willing to try to work at the relationship and go along together for counselling. But if your partner refuses to be involved, you may still want to get some help for yourself, so that you can assess where you are with the relationship, and decide how your own needs can best be met.

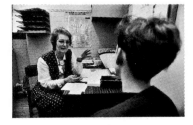

Leaving a relationship

Sadly, difficult and destructive relationships may be tolerated for years because of the apparent lack of alternatives, especially where women are financially dependent or have nowhere else to go, as is so often the case. There may be the very real fear that you will not be able to support yourself or your children. Or you may just feel paralysed by the difficulties you face.

Women caught up in difficult relationships may blame themselves in part, feeling that they have provoked or deserve the treatment they receive. It's difficult to feel good about yourself when you're in such a destructive relationship, and with self-esteem at rock bottom, it's harder to gather up the strength to do something about the situation. It may feel safer to stay in an unsatisfactory relationship, rather than face the emotional trauma and practical difficulties of leaving. Where there are dependent children, there may be additional pressures to stay for their sake, and guilt about the effect your problems may be having on them. Scary as it may feel, the best course of action may finally be to leave a difficult relationship, although this is seldom an easy choice to make.

Coping with loss

When a relationship with someone ends, for whatever reason, you will experience a sense of loss which will take time to adjust to. Whether the loss is owing to someone dying, a relationship breaking up, children or close friends moving away, even the loss of your job or your health, you may go through a similar process of coming to terms with the changes and adjusting to a new situation. Because our identity is often tied up closely with other people, the end of a relationship may leave us particularly vulnerable to stress and depression for which we need time and support.

Of course the pain you experience will depend a lot on the nature of your loss. While you may desperately miss your children when they leave home, this may be offset by your realisation that they need to find their own independence, and by new opportunities which open up for you. On the other hand, bereavement may be particularly traumatic because it is so final. Because women tend to live longer than men, it is common for them to experience the death of their husband or partner. The loss of a life-long and loving partner may be very hard to bear.

When a difficult relationship comes to an end, it can be an enormous relief. Suddenly, the restrictions that closed you in are lifted, the demands and violations gone, you can be your own person once more. But few relationships are all bad, and it takes time to adjust to being without the other person, however hard being with them was. There may well be feelings of guilt or sadness about the way things were, and you may still feel a sense of loss to do with the relationship ending.

'My husband was a really bad lot. When he left, I knew I was well rid of him. But he'd been a part of my life for thirty years, and he left a huge gap – I felt the loss terribly.'

When a relationship has not been open and visible to others, the loss you experience when it ends may be especially hard. If you are in a lesbian relationship and have chosen not to 'come out' or have not been accepted by family and friends, or are involved in an affair with someone who doesn't want the relationship revealed, your grief may well go unrecognised by those around you, leaving you with little support or comfort. It may help to find a close friend you can trust and confide in, or to seek professional counselling.

'When Jean died from breast cancer last year, I felt completely alone. Her family did all the arrangements for the funeral themselves, and didn't really want to acknowledge me at all. In the end, I decided to stay away just to keep the peace, but it hurt me terribly.'

There is no right way to grieve, but you will probably need a lot of support and time to come to terms with your loss. Commonly, people go through a number of different stages during the process of grieving, though how long each lasts and how severe it is will vary from one person to another. Numbness, shock and disbelief may be followed by a period of depression, grief or even anger. You may experience feelings of guilt, blaming yourself for the death or for things you might have done or said. Finally, you will come to accept your loss, and will be able to make some plans for the future.

Friends and family may believe they are helping by trying to cheer you up and stop you from thinking about your loss. In fact, what you need more than anything else is the chance to talk about your feelings and express your grief openly. It may help to talk to a bereavement counsellor – your doctor may be able to put you in touch with someone, or you could contact the voluntary organisation Cruse which provides advice and counselling to people who are coping with bereavement.

Stress

Why are women stressed?

Women have always been challenged by stressful lives. Today, more than ever before, many of us struggle to balance the different parts of our lives and cope with the many demands placed on us – shouldering the responsibility for home and children, caring for other family members, being denied many of the opportunities open to men, and feeling undervalued for what we do at home and at work. We work much longer hours than men, with less relaxation and time for ourselves. It's not surprising that many women identify stress as one of their main health problems.

While many women now enjoy a better standard of living, labour-saving devices and greater work opportunities, we continue to face enormous stresses. For women at home, housework is monotonous, isolating, and has no end – there's always something else to be done. It's also unpaid and low-status, making us financially dependent on a wage-earning partner or on benefits, and sometimes contributing to our feelings of low self-esteem. Women in paid work are most likely to be in low-paid, repetitive jobs, often part-time, with average earnings considerably less than those of men. Women in management and more senior positions often face the stress of having to prove themselves in a traditionally male environment. Working women usually also carry the main responsibility for home chores, whether or not they share that home with a man. Married women have been found to receive considerably less emotional support from their husbands than married men do from their wives which makes it harder to cope with problems.

Where there are dependent children, women play the major part in their care and upbringing and, if they work outside the home, it usually falls to them to take responsibility for arranging alternative childcare while they are at work, and hurrying home at the end of the day to spend 'quality' time with the children. Working mothers are the norm – the majority of mothers (67 per cent) with children over 5 and around a third of those with children under 5 are in paid employment.

We do everything we can to be effective in each area of our life – at work, with our partner, as mothers – and often this is at the expense of taking our own needs into account.

'My job became so important that it began to take over. I felt I had to give that bit more to prove my worth in a firm of architects where I was the only woman partner. I was staying late each evening, and taking work home every weekend. My life was out of balance . . .'

'Coping on my own with two young children, and holding down a part-time

job, I became more and more exhausted and run down. It was like running on a tread mill, and I was afraid to jump off for fear I'd never find the energy to get going again. There was never any time for me.'

How much stress is OK ?

It's impossible to avoid stress altogether, and a certain amount is positive – keeping you going and feeling alive. Some sources of stress are short-lived and can be coped with there and then – for example, going to the dentist, taking your driving test, or surviving Christmas! But too much stress can be bad for both physical and mental health. If the stress is long-term, like a destructive relationship or being out of work, then it's much more difficult to deal with and may be affecting your health.

People have different tolerance levels for stress. What is stimulating for one person may induce headaches, insomnia or other symptoms in another. How we react to a given situation will depend on our past experiences, our own inbuilt resilience and personality, and the sources of emotional support and material resources available. Certainly, having to cope with little money, poor housing conditions, or other aspects of poverty may well be a major source of stress in itself. And for black women, racism may also be a serious stress factor.

Sometimes we are unaware of the levels of stress we are under, because we are so used to them. It may actually hit us when we take a break and slow down, giving us a chance to reassess our day-to-day life. Or it may be that an otherwise small crisis which we would normally cope with, leads us to breaking point.

'I was under a lot of pressure at work – facing continuous harassment and under threat of redundancy – but I thought I was coping all right. Then the washing-machine broke down and flooded the kitchen – I just stood and screamed with all the pent-up frustration.'

How does your body react to stress?

When faced with a stressful situation, our bodies respond by preparing for some kind of action. The pituitary glands secrete the 'alarm' hormone ACTH, and this in turn causes the adrenal glands to secrete adrenaline, noradrenaline and cortisone hormones in what is called the 'fight or flight response'. Your pulse rate and breathing speed up, the pupils of your eyes dilate, your muscles tense and you may begin to sweat. Sugars and fatty acids are released from the liver into the blood to provide extra fuel for action. However, life in the nineties does not usually allow us to respond by fighting or running away. With no natural outlet to deal with the physiological changes of the stress response, we tend to internalise feelings of anxiety, anger or frustration. Women are particularly likely to bottle these feelings up, because it's less acceptable for us to express anger or frustration in the ways which men commonly do. Over time, this may contribute to a number of different health problems, including high blood pressure, indigestion, ulcers, migraine, asthma, irritable bowel syndrome, back pain and skin complaints, reduced immune system effectiveness, and heart disease – quite a catalogue of ill health!

Are you stressed?

Getting to know the particular danger signs that indicate you are under too much stress will mean you can respond quickly, both to try to remove or reduce some of the causes, and to put some of your coping strategies into practice. Be aware of some of the more harmful coping mechanisms you may be tempted to use, such as smoking, drinking or over-eating. A very stressful period may not be the best time to try to do something about these if you have come to rely on them, but being aware of them and looking for alternative ways of coping will help you to keep them under control until you can tackle them more seriously.

Everyone reacts differently, but you may experience one or more of these if you are suffering from stress:

- not being able to get to sleep or waking early
- moodiness and irritability
- lack of appetite or over-eating
- nail-biting and teeth-grinding
- being wound up
- shouting and slamming doors
- being obsessive
- tightness in chest and chest pains
- being indecisive
- loss of interest in sex

If you are worried by any symptoms, you should talk to your doctor. But there are also things you can do for yourself to begin to reduce the amount of stress you have to deal with, and to cope better with the stress you can't avoid.

Making life less stressful

To make your life less stressful and to help you cope with stresses that you can't avoid, it's helpful to think ahead. You may not be particularly stressed just now, but things can change unexpectedly – bereavement, a new job, someone ill in the family – and having some coping strategies at hand will help you through a difficult time. Start by identifying several of the key areas of stress in your life, and place them into the four different categories in the diagram to see how well in balance you are.

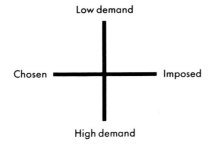

Make a list of all the low-demand stresses which you feel you can do something about. Sometimes this is just a question of making choices and saying no or compromising over certain things. Try to be more realistic about what you can achieve in the time you have, and make sure you build in some time for yourself. Opt for a take-away or 'pot-luck' rather than preparing an elaborate meal for friends; be less fussy about the housework while you are coping with the demands of a new baby; and delegate as much as you can rather than trying to do everything yourself.

Areas of stress which you have actually chosen are probably the easiest to deal with because they are likely to provide pleasure, serve a purpose or offer some other benefits to offset some of the stress they cause! The chosen and demanding areas may well be some of the things which stretch you and give you satisfaction and a sense of achievement. Although stressful, the pay-off may well be worthwhile in terms of fulfilment or increased opportunities. Studying for a new qualification or learning a new skill, having a baby or taking on some extra responsibility at work are all possible examples of these types of stress. Too many of these stresses at one time may overwhelm you, leaving you too anxious and worn out to enjoy the positive side, so where you have a choice it's important not to take on too many demands at one time.

The stresses that are imposed on you may well be the most difficult to cope with and the most difficult to do something about. They are likely to have the least to offer in the way of positive benefits. Where they serve a useful purpose for others, there may be a good deal of resistance to changes you try to introduce. Being caught up in a violent or otherwise destructive relationship, caring for a dependent relative, or having an unrewarding job with long hours and low pay are examples of these types of stress. Being ill or incapacitated yourself can also lead to high levels of stress – again, it's because you are not in control.

'With my leg in plaster, I suddenly became completely helpless and dependent on others. I couldn't drive, in fact I couldn't get out of the house at all. I hated having to ask for help, and got terribly frustrated not being able to get on with things myself. My blood pressure soared sky-high.'

We all have a certain amount of stress imposed on us, but we need to be careful that the balance doesn't tip too far in this direction. These may be some of the most challenging areas for us to confront. We need to find support from others to help make necessary changes. A step-by-step approach may be best, starting with small practical changes and working towards bigger solutions. You may not be able to change a relationship overnight, but you could talk to your partner about how you are feeling and lay down some boundaries for acceptable behaviour; although there may be no easy solutions to the demands of caring, you could think through what you are not prepared to do, and negotiate with other family members to share some of the burden.

Depression

What is depression?

Depression is one of those terms which is used to describe a wide range of feelings or situations, some of them very trivial. What most of us refer to as depression – when we feel miserable and want to be left alone for a while – is really just a low mood which is usually triggered off by some specific problem and passes fairly quickly. Because of the casual way in which the word is used, depression may not be taken as seriously as a more obvious condition such as a broken arm or pneumonia. There may be a tendency to be unsympathetic, blaming the person for the way they are and expecting them to snap out of it.

Unlike the transient low moods that most of us experience from time to time, clinical depression is a physical phenomenon, with symptoms lasting for two weeks or more. It is caused by the neurotransmitters in the brain, particularly noradrenaline and serotonin. These chemicals are secreted by millions of nerve-endings and they affect the capacity of the brain cells to send messages to each other in the area that controls sleep, appetite, sexual desire and mood. Clinical depression occurs when the neurotransmitters fail to work effectively. The brain becomes like a car engine with a flat battery. This is why although we usually associate depression with extreme misery, sadness or despair, most people suffering from clinical depression describe themselves as feeling numb, flat, listless, detached and unable to take an interest in anything. The distinction is important.

'I lost interest in everything I'd ever enjoyed and became a total recluse. Some evenings I couldn't even bother to turn on the TV – I'd just sit and wait for it to be bedtime. Even though I was lethargic, I felt constantly anxious and tense, always on the verge of tears.'

If you or someone you know is suffering from clinical depression, you may notice one or more of the following signs. Unfortunately, the more depressed you become, the more likely you are to fail to notice the signs, or do nothing about them, but if you suffer from any of these for more than a week or two you should seek help:

- change in sleep patterns (you can't get to sleep, wake early or want to sleep all the time)
- loss or gain of appetite or weight
- unexplained tiredness
- loss of concentration, memory, or ability to make decisions
- being agitated or slowed down
- loss of self-confidence and low self-esteem
- suicidal thoughts

It's easy for women to feel guilty if they are not coping with everyday life, but it's important to recognise that clinical depression is an illness, that you are not to blame for feeling the way you do, and that you may need help to overcome the problem. There is an enormous stigma attached to mental health problems which may make it harder for us to face up to our situation and seek help. Other people's lack of understanding can be one of the worst things to bear.

Why do women get depressed?

Depression is particularly common among women. Twice as many women as men complain of depression, perhaps because they are more willing to take their problems to a doctor, while men may be more likely to turn to other sources of refuge such as drink. It's also likely that women have more cause to become depressed, having more stress, hardship and isolation and less control over their lives. There is also a strong link between depression and poverty, and women are more likely to have a low income.

Depression may be a response to specific events or problems. It is often associated with loss such as bereavement, redundancy or divorce. A period of depression is a perfectly normal and appropriate response to such an event. You may need the chance to talk through your problem with a friend, or get professional counselling to help you through a stressful or difficult period. Sometimes we find that depression may develop without any obvious cause or event to trigger it. This can make it harder for others to accept and for you to understand, and treatment may be more difficult.

Some medical experts believe that tendencies towards depression are shaped in early life by our parents and by childhood events. There seems to be a link with low self-esteem which in turn stems from the way we are treated when we are young.

Depression often runs in families, and it seems that you are more likely to suffer from depression if your parents did, though it is likely that depressive behaviour is learnt rather than being inherited. We know that children tend to copy the behaviour of their parents, for example, a child growing up with violent parents is more likely to resort to violence because it is seen as an acceptable response to certain situations.

Are you at risk ?

Research has shown that some women are more at risk of becoming seriously depressed than others. You are more likely to be prone to depression if any of the following apply to you:

- you have pre-school children
- you have three or more children under 14 living at home
- you have a low income
- you do not do paid work outside the home
- you do not have an intimate relationship to provide support
- you have suffered a loss or bereavement early in life (especially if you lost your mother before the age of 11)

Obviously, not everyone in these situations will get depressed – in fact, it sometimes seems remarkable that more women are not depressed, considering the stresses and strains which they face. A variety of factors may help to buffer the effects of the above, including the kind of emotional support and financial resources available to you, your personality and your upbringing.

Women may be particularly prone to depression at certain times, and some people believe that this is owing to changing hormone levels. While this may be true in part, there may well be other factors and it's wrong to assume that women are entirely the victims of their hormones.

Premenstrual syndrome

Premenstrual Syndrome (PMS) includes a number of different symptoms, but some women with PMS do feel low and depressed during the days before their period. Hormonal imbalances are probably responsible for mood changes, though not all women are sensitive to them. (For more on PMS, see pages 46-51.)

Menopause

Similarly, during the years leading up to the menopause, fluctuating levels of hormones may cause some women to feel low or depressed. However, there may be other changes that are just as likely to be the cause of any depression you experience.

Post-natal depression

Most women experience the 'baby-blues', feeling weepy and irritable in the first two or three days after childbirth. This is quite normal and soon passes. It may be owing to hormonal changes which occur shortly after delivery, and to the enormous emotional upheaval and adjustments that come with having a new baby.

For around one in ten new mothers, a more serious depression develops some time during the first few months after childbirth. Post-natal depression is one of the most common complications of childbirth in the Western world, and around half of the women affected will need help to get through it. You may feel weepy, unable to cope and inadequate as a mother. It helps to be able to talk about your feelings to someone close, or to someone who has been through a similar experience. Your health visitor or GP will also offer help and support, and treatment where necessary.

'I coped very well at first, but then I began to feel more and more out of control. I felt the baby was sucking the energy out of me. I couldn't sleep. I felt permanently irritated, grouchy and resentful. I was also very frightened by my feelings. Sometimes I would listen to the baby crying and crying and couldn't bring myself to go to him. It was as though he was someone else's child. I wanted him to be someone else's responsibility. I hated his dependence on me. People kept saying that all new mothers felt strange, but I couldn't believe this was normal. One day I actually left him *in his pram outside the supermarket and started to walk home. That's when I realised I needed help.'*

Getting Help for Mental Health Problems

Doing something about a problem early on can make it easier. It may be that the way to improve our mental health is to change the situation – find friends, start a new job, move house, or end a caring role – or we may need to get help from our doctor. Unfortunately, a lot of mental illness goes undetected in the GP's surgery, leading to inappropriate treatment or referral. Many GPs are getting better at recognising depression and offering effective treatment, and there are a number of treatment options available.

Counselling

The counsellor will help you think through the difficulties you are facing and jointly you can work out ways of dealing with them.

Psychotherapies

A range of effective psychotherapies has been developed to treat different mental health problems. Cognitive and interpersonal therapies are particularly useful for treating depression and eating disorders; others include behaviourial therapies and family therapy. Your GP should be able to refer you for therapy.

Drug treatment

There are more tranquillisers and anti-depressants prescribed in the UK than any other drug, and they are mostly prescribed to women. There is now a new generation of effective drugs, especially anti-psychotics and anti-depressants, but they need to be used with care. While a short course of drug treatment may be useful in helping you through difficult times, effectiveness decreases over time, and the drug may mask underlying symptoms of depression which may then remain untreated. The drugs may actually make it harder for you to identify or tackle the root cause of your problems. You may experience side-effects – drowsiness and tiredness are common, although it is sometimes difficult to distinguish the symptoms of the original condition from the side-effects. After taking drugs for a lengthy period, you may find it difficult to come off them or to reduce the dose, possibly experiencing unpleasant or alarming withdrawal symptoms.

It is now recognised that many tranquillisers are addictive, and you need to be wary of using them over too long a period. If your GP suggests that you take a tranquilliser, check exactly what kind of tablets are being offered, and how they will help you. Find out about any possible side-effects, and whether you can have other medicines or alcohol while you are taking them. Be sure to find out how long you may need to continue with them, and when you should see your doctor again. Certainly beware if your doctor offers repeat prescriptions without seeing you to talk about your progress.

If you are worried that you may be addicted to tranquillisers or other medication, see the addresses at the end of the book.

Hypnotherapy

This can be useful in helping you come off tranquillisers, or cope with depression and anxiety. While it doesn't work for everyone, it can produce faster relief than other treatments. Your GP will be able to refer you to a reputable hypnotist.

Always check the qualifications of a hypnotherapist before you make an appointment.

Taking Care of Mental Health

The following strategies all offer ways to reduce your risk of mental health problems, enhancing your family and social relationships, improving your performance in the things you do, and increasing your productivity and creativity. It helps to consider positive ways to respond to stresses rather than becoming overwhelmed by them. Finding ways of coping and feeling more in control makes it easier to face up to and tackle any problems.

Assertiveness

Assertiveness means recognising that you are valuable in your own right, and that your needs and desires are valid. Being assertive allows you to act in your own best interests and stand up for your rights while also respecting the rights and feelings of others. It helps you to express both positive and negative feelings comfortably, to ask for what you want, to say no and to set limits. Being more assertive may help you avoid some stressful situations, and cope better with others. Assertiveness will allow you to be confident about telling people what you want, without being threatening or putting them down. Remember it's OK to change your mind, negotiate, or say no and you don't have to feel guilty. Being assertive means people will believe you when you say no or tell them how you feel, especially if you match your body language to what you are saying.

Sometimes people confuse assertiveness with aggression – but they are quite different. Aggressive behaviour is when you try to get what you want at any cost, with no thought or feeling for others. It can involve putting other people down, bullying, being sarcastic, using emotional blackmail or flattery.

Being assertive is not just about how you deal with other people, but also about how you feel about yourself and talk to yourself. You may be your own worst enemy, telling yourself that you are no good at something or that you ought to put everyone else first. Try not to doubt yourself or feel small. Think positive and believe in your own value. It's all too easy to find yourself justifying your actions or feelings, succumbing to pressure from family and friends, or avoiding conflict by not challenging others. (See How you see yourself, pages 8-9.)

'I just kept telling myself that I could do it, it would be all right. Everyone said I was mad to go in for a degree course at my age, but I knew it was what I wanted. It was a marvellous feeling when I graduated – I felt I'd proved myself.'

It may help to think through some situations where you need to become more assertive. What might happen if you do assert yourself? Do you have too much to lose? Initially, the people around you may react badly if they aren't used to your being assertive. Your family and friends may accuse you of being awkward, or your partner may complain because he or she has a vested interest in your staying the way you are. You may need to take things step by step, making a few changes at a time. Think of what you'll gain as you become more assertive. You will be able to:

- say what you want
- put your own needs first
- stand up to the prejudices of others
- say no without feeling guilty
- say what you mean and mean what you say
- give and receive compliments and criticism
- set limits to what you are prepared to do or accept
- feel more in control, and get rid of all that guilt

If you feel you need to develop some skills in assertiveness, you could find out about groups or classes – these may be available at adult education centres, or privately. You could do more reading about some of the techniques. It's really a question of practising and trying out different approaches, and developing your confidence as you discover that it makes a difference to the way you feel!

Physical activity

Taking some kind of regular physical activity can help if you are feeling stressed, and may protect you from becoming depressed. And if you are feeling low, exercise can actually help lift your mood. This is probably through the action of endorphins – hormone-like chemicals released when you exercise which produce a feeling of well-being. The sense of achievement you may feel from having motivated yourself to do something positive will also probably help to raise your self-esteem and make you feel good. (For more about physical activity, see pages 192-211.)

Relaxation

Relaxation is essential for our health. Our many conflicting roles today put us under more pressure than ever before. A woman in the nineties is expected to be an efficient worker, caring mother, intelligent friend and partner and exciting lover. If you feel you need a split personality and a thirty-hour day to achieve everything you have to do, remember you're not alone.

Relaxation is valuable for coping with all the pressure. It can help relieve stress, tension, high blood pressure, and pain, for example during childbirth, and can be useful in helping you give up smoking or other dependent habits such as tranquilliser use.

It's easy to learn different relaxation techniques, but the important part is making sure you incorporate them into your day-to-day life – that way you will very quickly begin to feel the benefit.

Time for yourself

Being short of time and doing everything at breakneck speed is a major cause of stress, and not having time to relax makes it harder to cope with stress. It helps to learn some simple relaxation skills and build them into your everyday life. Get to know some of the things that help you relax – time with friends, time on your own, massage, a lazy bath, physical activity – and plan to make time for some of them each day. Prioritise the things you have to do, and try not to set unrealistic goals. Don't feel bad about taking short cuts or saying no to certain requests or expectations placed on you. Instead, make time for things that you want to do. The following suggestions will help you feel calmer and less stressed:

- do one thing at a time
- listen without interrupting
- escape into tasks that demand concentration
- eat slowly and savour food
- find a private retreat at home
- plan some relaxation each day
- avoid hurry whenever possible.

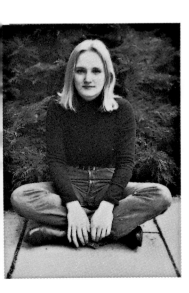

Often women think of time to relax as an optional extra – something to enjoy when everything else is done, if there's time – but in fact it's as essential to your health as eating well and getting enough activity. Try to set aside at least half an hour each day where you stop everything you have to do, and do something you want to do. It may seem strange at first – almost selfish! – to find even such a small amount of time. But actually you will simply be giving yourself the minimum amount of relaxation which you need to keep going and keep well.

If you can't switch off from your problems because worries crowd into your mind, spend the time on something that crowds them out – reading is great for this, or chatting with a friend. If you feel physically tense, something active may be the best way to work it out of your system. The feelings of jittery anxiety which you experience when you're tense are caused by an over-production of noradrenaline – the fight or flight hormone. When this happens, it helps to burn it up in the way in which nature intended. You may not be able to run away from your problem, but a brisk walk, swim or workout or any other physical activity will literally work the hormones out of your system, leaving you feeling more relaxed.

Quick release of tension

Learning to breathe slowly and gently is useful for when you feel anxious, panicky or uptight, and may help if you have trouble getting to sleep. It's a good way of coping with a possibly stressful situation such as having an internal examination or going into an interview.

- let your breath go (don't breathe in first)
- take in a slow gentle breath, and hold it for a second
- let it go with a leisurely sigh of relief
- drop your shoulders at the same time and relax your hands
- make sure your teeth are not clenched together
- if you have to speak, speak more slowly in a lower tone of voice

5-minute relaxation

You can use this technique whenever you have only a short time to spare. It's better if you have a chair with arms, but you should be able to learn to relax anywhere you find yourself – at home, at work, on the bus. Use a cushion in the small of your back if this helps, and make sure you are warm and not likely to be disturbed.

1   Sit upright and well back in the chair so that your thighs and back are supported, and rest your hands in the cradle position on your lap, or

lightly on top of your thighs. If you like, take off your shoes, and let your feet rest on the ground (if they don't touch the floor, try to find a book or similar object to rest them on). If you want to, close your eyes.

2   Begin by breathing out first. Then breathe in easily, just as much as you need. Now breathe out slowly, with a slight sigh, like a balloon slowly deflating. Do this once more, slowly . . . breathe in . . . breathe out . . . as you breathe out, feel the tension begin to drain away. Then go back to your ordinary breathing: even, quiet, steady.

3   Now direct your thoughts to each part of your body in turn, to the muscles and joints.

- Think first about your left foot. Your toes are still. Your foot feels heavy on the floor. Let your foot and toes start to feel completely relaxed.
- Now think about your right foot . . . toes . . . ankles . . . they are resting heavily on the floor. Let both your feet, your toes, ankles start to relax.
- Now think about your legs. Let your legs feel completely relaxed and heavy on the chair. Your thighs, your knees roll downwards when they relax, so let them go.
- Think now about your back, and your spine. Let the tension drain away from your back, and from your spine. Follow your breathing, and each time you breathe out, relax your back and spine a little more.
- Let your abdominal muscles become soft and loose. There's no need to hold your stomach in tight, it rises and falls as you breathe quietly – feel that your stomach is completely relaxed.
- No tension in your chest. Let your breathing be slow and easy, and each time your breathe out, let go a little more.
- Think now about the fingers of your left hand – they are curved, limp and quite still. Now the fingers of your right hand . . . relaxed . . . soft and still. Let this feeling of relaxation spread – up your arms . . . feel the heaviness in your arms up to your shoulders. Let your shoulders relax, let them drop easily . . . and then let them drop even further than you thought they could.

- Think about your neck. Feel the tension melt away from your neck and shoulders. Each time you breathe out, relax your neck a little more.

- Now before we move on, just check to see if all these parts of your body are still relaxed – your feet, legs, back and spine, tummy, hands, arms, neck and shoulders. Keep your breathing gentle and easy. Every time you breathe out, relax a little more, and let all the tensions ease away from your body. No tensions . . . just enjoy this feeling of relaxation.

- Now think about your face. Let the expression come off your face. Smooth out your brow and let your forehead feel wide and relaxed. Let your eyebrows drop gently. There's no tension round your eyes . . . your eyelids slightly closed, your eyes are still. Let your jaw unwind . . . teeth slightly apart as your jaw unwinds more and more. Feel the relief of letting go.

- Now think about your tongue, and throat. Let your tongue drop down to the bottom of your mouth and relax completely. Relax your tongue and throat. And your lips . . . lips lightly together, no pressure between them.

- Let all your muscles in your face unwind and let go – there's no tension in your face – just let it relax more and more.

4   Now, instead of thinking about yourself in parts, feel the all-over sensation of letting go, of quiet and of rest. Check to see if you are still relaxed. Stay like this for a few moments, and listen to your breathing . . . in . . . and out . . . let your body become looser, heavier, each time you breathe out.

5   Now continue for a little longer, and enjoy this time for relaxation.

6   Coming back – slowly, wriggle your hands a little, and your feet. When you are ready, open your eyes and sit quietly for a while. Stretch, if you want to, or yawn, and slowly start to move again.

If you find it hard to practise this relaxation technique on your own, or want a little more guidance, there are relaxation tapes and books available, or you might join a group with an experienced teacher to help you. You could try your health centre or adult education centre to see what they offer.

Meditation

Meditation is a way of relaxing the mind. Your heart rate and breathing slow down as your need for oxygen reduces, and you feel calm and relaxed. There are different ways to meditate, but one of the simplest is to focus your mind on one particular sound or picture, thereby removing everyday thoughts and worries.

Once you get used to meditating, try to practise every day – morning and evening is ideal if only you can make the time. Find a warm, quiet place where you won't be disturbed – if that sounds impossible, you could lock yourself in the bathroom or let your family know that you need a bit of time to yourself! Make sure you are breathing slowly and gently. Close your eyes and choose an image to think about – some flowers, a garden, the sea – or decide on a sound, for example 'one', and say it to yourself every time you breathe out. If everyday thoughts come into your mind to disturb you, just note them mentally and then let them pass, and bring your mind back to what you are focusing on. You can continue for a few minutes at first, but gradually you will be able to build up to about twenty minutes. When you are ready, slowly wriggle your hands and feet a little, open your eyes, and sit quietly for a while. Stretch if you want or yawn, and slowly start to move again.

Massage

Massage can be a good way to relax, bringing immediate relief from headaches and muscle tension, and offering a useful therapy for both physical and emotional problems, such as PMS and depression. Combining it with the use of aromatic oils can make it even more effective (see Aromatherapy, page 316). Make sure you have a warm room, and plenty of time so you don't have to hurry.

Self-massage

- Self-massage is a technique you can use whenever you like to help relieve obstinate muscle tension or pain, or before loosening exercises or relaxation. Think of it as 'oiling' the joints and muscles to ease them into movement and stimulate the blood supply. Massage should be rhythmical and the pressure varied according to what feels good. Relax both your hands and keep them as loose and flexible as possible when you are moving them.

- Shoulders – hand on opposite shoulder, roll the back muscle up and forward.
- Neck – thumbs along the edge of skull from ears towards spine; change to fingers and continue down spine; then push the back neck muscles up towards head.
- Forehead – for 'vertical wrinkles' – start at centre of forehead, stroke rhythmically out and down to ears. For 'horizontal wrinkles' – stroke from eyebrows to hairline, each hand in turn.
- Eyes – 'palming' – close your eyes and place the palms of your hands, one over each eyesocket. Let your fingers cross over your forehead. The resulting darkness is very restful.
- Lips – with fingertips massage lips over teeth.
- Scalp – 'hair washing' – moving scalp over skull with fingertips.
- For sinus pain – with fingertips gently massage over site of pain.

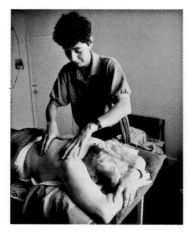

You could share a massage with your partner, or a friend. It can be a marvellous way of relaxing together, and can make you feel especially close. You don't have to remove clothes if you don't feel comfortable with this. Feet, head and neck massages may be good ones to start with. Apply pressure and don't be nervous about hurting the other person – you can always check with them. Mould your hands to fit the contours over which they are passing, and try not to break contact with the skin until you have finished, to help keep the continuity of feeling. Feel centred and relaxed about the way you are standing, sitting or kneeling. You may also find that massaging a friend helps you to relax as well.

With a friend

Forehead massage
This is very useful for relieving headaches and tension.

- Hold palms against the forehead for a few moments. Cover the forehead with the hands, let the fingers spread. Apply no pressure. Pause as long as it seems OK – let your friend grow used to your touch. Centre yourself and make sure you feel relaxed – focus on your breathing if this helps.
- Now begin to massage the forehead with the balls of your thumbs. First, mentally divide the forehead into strips about half an inch wide. Start with your thumbs at the centre of the forehead just below the hairline – glide both thumbs at once in either direction outwards along the top-most strip. Continue towards the temples, and end there by moving your thumbs in a circle about half an inch wide.
- Then, without taking your hands off the forehead, return to the centre of the forehead and begin again – the next strip down.
- Work progressively down – ending with a circle on the temples – to the last strip just above your friend's eyebrows. This is the first stage of complete face massage.
Variation: two hands on the forehead, smooth one back from eyebrows over the scalp and then the other.

Neck and shoulders
Stand behind your friend, put your hands on her shoulders and centre yourself so that you feel comfortable.

- Place your hands on your friend's shoulders with your thumbs at the back. Use your thumbs in small circular movements – work up from the top of the spine to the hairline – slowly. With each circular motion, try to feel aware of the tension and to work it away. Hold your whole hand in contact with her shoulders, and although you're concentrating on the neck, be aware of tension in the shoulders too, and try to work that away.

- Then try in any way that feels right to you, to smooth away tension in her neck and shoulders.
- To end, press down with the hands on top of the shoulders and then let the hands travel down the upper arms as far as the elbows. Repeat this a few times.

Foot massage

This is wonderfully soothing! We often neglect our feet, hate them, think they are too ugly or smelly! It's good to give them a treat. Your friend can lie down, or sit with her foot on a stool.

- Massage the sole of the foot with the tips of your thumbs. Press hard, as if you were putting a drawing pin into a piece of wood. Press everywhere. Work slowly over the sole.
- Then lift the foot slightly and work the sides of the heel all the way to the ankle bone. Try to feel as if you are pushing away all the tension. Stop if it hurts, and change position.
- You can then work on the toes, and the top of the foot in the same way.

Yoga

Yoga can benefit both the mind and the body, involving the use of both posture and breathing exercises, which in turn can help with meditation. It can be effective in relieving stress and tension, and has been shown to be valuable in reducing blood pressure and pulse rate, and improving suppleness and joint movement. Yoga can be especially useful during pregnancy, improving posture and so alleviating backache and other aches and pains, and offering useful breathing exercises to help you relax and cope with the birth.

In order to learn yoga, you need to go along to a class or find someone to teach you. Adult education centres and sports and leisure centres often offer classes for beginners upwards. Once you have learnt some of the postures and breathing exercises, you will be able to practise at home in your own time.

T'ai Chi

This form of exercise originated in China, and involves slow, gentle flowing actions which makes it suitable for everyone – even people who are unable to do more strenuous exercise. Like yoga, it combines movement and breathing exercises with meditation. T'ai Chi exercises every part of the body, and has been said to improve flexibility and strength and to reduce the risk of osteoporosis, hardening of the arteries, tension, anger, depression and tiredness.

To find out about classes in your area, contact your local adult education centre (in the phone book).

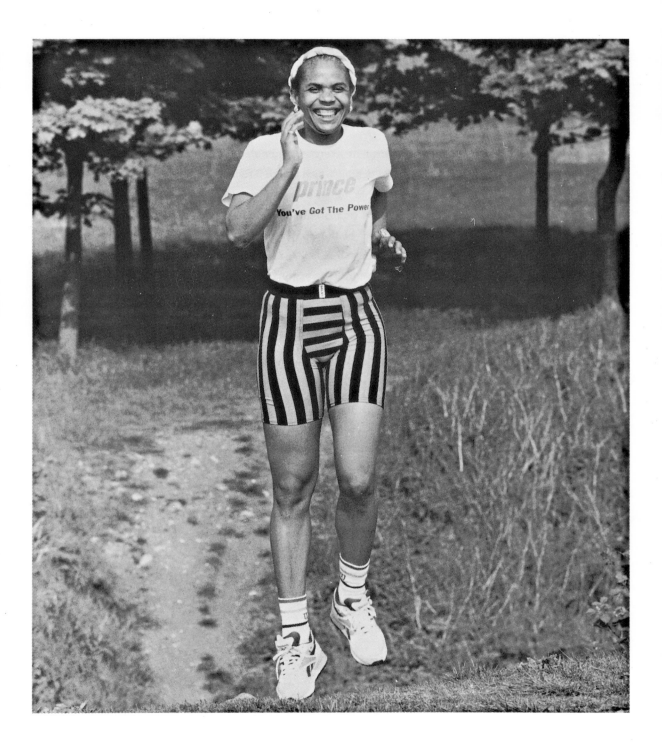

Your Reproductive Cycle

Throughout each month our bodies are in a state of change. From day to day different hormones surge forward and recede. Unless a woman is using a hormonal method of contraception, like the pill, her reproductive system is constantly at work building up to the release of an egg, trying to create the most suitable environment for fertilisation, thickening and enriching the lining of the womb ready to receive a fertilised egg and then, if no such egg implants, triggering the release of the womb lining (endometrium) ready to begin the process all over again.

The hormone levels in men vary too, but not on a day-to-day basis. In men, levels of testosterone and other reproductive hormones surge when they reach peak fertility in their late-teens, then they decline very, very slowly. But there is no great change from one day to the next. On average men start producing sperm when they are 13 and from then until they are well into old age, sperm are made at the rate of about 1,000 per second in each testicle, day and night.

A woman, on the other hand, is born with a lifetime's supply of potential eggs already in her ovaries. At six months' gestation a female foetus has a million or so potential eggs, and the number gradually diminishes, after birth and throughout childhood, until by the time she reaches puberty there are about 300,000 immature eggs (or oocytes) stored in her two ovaries. From before she starts her periods, from even before she is born, these immature eggs ripen and die on a cyclical basis.

When most young women reach the ages of 12 or 13 they begin to experience their reproductive cycle in an obvious way: their periods start.

We often think of our period as being at the end of our cycle. But in fact with the first day of your period a new cycle is already beginning. The cycle starts in the brain. On the first day of menstruation the part of the brain that controls basic bodily functions like hunger and thirst (the hypothalamus) releases a special hormone known as Luteinizing Hormone - Releasing Hormone (LH-RH). This hormone delivers a special chemical message to the pituitary gland at the base of the brain telling it to start manufacturing another hormone known as Follicle Stimulating Hormone (FSH). FSH seeps into your blood stream and makes its way to your ovaries where it gives the signal for hundreds of follicles (small balls of cells with an unripe egg in the middle) to start to grow and ripen.

For reasons that no one has yet discovered, one follicle always responds better to the FSH than the others and surges ahead. As it ripens the other follicles die back. As the single follicle ripens it produces large amounts of the hormone oestrogen which is absorbed into the blood stream. This oestrogen stimulates the cervix, the neck of the womb, to start producing wet stretchy mucus. The lining of the womb also picks up signals from the oestrogen and starts to thicken from 0.5 mm to around 7mm, to provide a rich, nourishing environment for a fertilised egg.

The oestrogen travels to the brain where it tells the pituitary gland to shut off its production of FSH and start producing another hormone called Luteinizing Hormone, or LH. The LH travels in the blood to the ovaries where the follicle is now bulging (it is the size of a pea) from the surface of the ovary. When it feels the LH around it the follicle bursts and releases its tiny egg. This part of the process is known as ovulation. In the day leading up to ovulation around one woman in ten experiences a tenderness or cramping known as Mittelschmerz (middle pain).

2.1 Egg released from ovary

Although the egg is the largest cell in a woman's body, it is smaller than a grain of salt. When it is released from the follicle it drops into the reach of the feathery fronds at the end of the fallopian tube. The fallopian tube is filled with tiny hair-like projections which waft the egg along. While the egg is making its journey down towards the womb, the empty follicle, which is now known as the corpus luteum, begins to release a new hormone, progesterone. This gives the womb lining a signal to make final preparations for a fertilised egg. On receiving the message it begins to store sugar and proteins in its spongy thick lining. The raised progesterone level also instructs the cervix to stop producing sperm-friendly wet mucus and start making thick mucus again. It also orders the pituitary gland to stop producing LH or FSH.

If the egg is fertilised it sends chemical signals to the corpus luteum to continue pumping out progesterone. If the egg is not fertilised the progesterone production eases. Deprived of a constant supply of progesterone, the womb lining begins to break down and the womb begins to contract to its pre-engorged size as the stored blood oozes away through the vagina as your period. As soon as the pituitary gland realises that the production of progesterone has stopped it starts pumping out FSH and the whole cycle starts all over again.

The fluctuating levels of hormones can be experienced by your body in ways that do not seem obviously connected to your reproductive cycle.

Before menstruation, the rising level of progesterone may cause your breasts to swell and your nipples to feel tender. You may find that your weight increases (sometimes by as much as 2 or 3 pounds) and you may feel bloated. This is mainly owing to fluid retention and you may find you urinate less.

During menstruation your metabolic rate, the rate at which you burn up calories, accelerates and some women find they crave foods high in carbohydrates such as pasta or chocolate. You may find you need to urinate more often to release that retained fluid.

Between your period and ovulation you may find that you are more prone to spots and, as you approach ovulation, your temperature rises slightly and your weight may increase a little, although the amount of

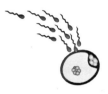

2.2 Egg being fertilised

2.3 Fertilised egg dividing

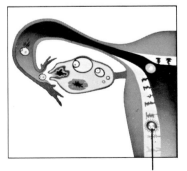

2.4 Egg implanting in womb lining

chloresterol in your blood lowers by a fraction. Some women find that their sensitivity to smell increases and many find that their libido increases.

Some doctors believe that the constantly fluctuating levels of hormones in our bodies may increase our risk of reproductive cancers. It seems to be the case that women with suppressed ovulation (for example, women using a hormonal method of contraception) have a reduced risk of cancer of the ovaries which is one of the most common cancers found in young women. Almost two-thirds of sufferers die from the disease within five years of diagnosis. A woman who has been on the pill for five years reduces her risk of ovarian cancer by 60 per cent. Pill users are also half as likely to suffer cancer of the womb lining. Doctors are not entirely sure why this is, but it has been suggested that our bodies simply are not designed to cope with repeated ovulation month after month.

Premenstrual Syndrome

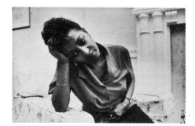

Most of us suffer symptoms that indicate that a period is due, but these affect all of us differently. In some women premenstrual symptoms are barely noticeable, but others suffer dreadfully.

'Before my periods my breasts swell up so much I have a bra two cup-sizes larger than the one I wear during the rest of the month. They feel really tender too, and hurt if I have to run. The day before I start, my lower back feels stiff and my stomach feels really bloated. It's hard to put my finger on it but I just feel horrible.'

'During the week before my period I get more spotty than usual – especially on my back and chest. All week I get odd grumbling pains in my stomach, not cramps, just an ache. I used to start cramping a couple of hours before I started to bleed and that was a good warning sign, now I sometimes start bleeding before the cramps!'

'It sounds strange but my husband seems to notice my premenstrual symptoms more than I do. He says my stomach and my breasts swell and that my body smell changes slightly. He even told me once that he thought I was going to start my period early, and I did!'

'When I read about premenstrual problems I think I must be unique because I actually feel better before my period. My spotty skin clears up and I feel more alert.'

'The two days before each period starts is murder for my whole family. In fact sometimes I'm surprised I haven't literally killed someone. I don't get any of the bad pains you hear about – I just seem to go to pieces. I turn into a real fumble-fingers, I drop and spill everything I touch. I forget everything, and I tend to burst into tears at the slightest excuse – even if I watch something sad on the news.'

All these women have very different premenstrual experiences, but they are all quite normal. Only about 10 per cent of women have no premenstrual symptoms at all and as many as 30 per cent of us are driven to seek medical help from a doctor. Five women in every 100 are completely incapacitated and have to take time off work.

For some women premenstrual syndrome is good news. American researchers in Seattle and San Francisco found that 25 per cent of women reported premenstrual bursts of energy, increased feelings of sexual desire and a general sense of well-being. But for most of us the days before our period can be the darkest in the month.

Doctors disagree about exactly why some women suffer and others escape. Some think it's a direct reaction to the changes in the balance of hormones at this time. Others maintain that there is a strong psychological component, arguing that even when women's cycles are altered (for example when they are on the pill), they still complain of symptoms. Still

Common Premenstrual Symptoms

More than 150 premenstrual symptoms have been described. The following are the most common.

Physical

- stomach cramps
- backache
- headache
- muscle stiffness
- swolen, tender breasts
- sore nipples
- water retention
- weight gain
- tiredness

Psychological

- tension
- irritability
- anger
- depression
- anxiety
- mood swings
- tearfulness
- increased/lowered sex drive
- food cravings
- sleeplessness

others dispute that it exists at all. Some specialists believe that the term 'Premenstrual Syndrome' is used to cover such a huge range of symptoms, in such varying intensity, needing such different treatments, that the term is useless.

The medical disagreements over the cause and nature of premenstrual syndrome can sometimes make it difficult to get medical help, especially if your doctor maintains that it is 'all in the mind'. However, the majority of the medical establishment has come round to the view that there is, without doubt, 'a set of emotional, behavioural and physical symptoms that recur regularly during the second half of each menstrual cycle, with complete absence of symptoms after menstruation' (Drug and Therapeutics Bulletin 1992 vol 30 no 18 – an update sent out to all doctors). In short, premenstrual syndrome officially exists!

If you keep a chart of how your cycle affects your life (see page 61), you will easily see the cluster of pre-period symptoms that indicate premenstrual syndrome. If you visit your GP for advice or help about premenstrual syndrome, he or she will probably ask you to chart your symptoms for at least two months. By already doing so, you can speed up the diagnostic process.

If your premenstrual syndrome is severe, there are drugs that your GP can prescribe. However, some doctors may be reluctant to do so if they are not convinced that they will be effective. 'Doubting doctors' are not simply being difficult. In trials where some women have been given a drug, but others have been given a placebo – a substance which medically would have no effect whatsoever – more than half the women taking the placebo have reported relief from symptoms. In one trial using surgically inserted hormonal implants 94 per cent of the women receiving empty implants said they felt much better.

The following drug treatments are available. If your premenstrual symptoms are severe enough to disrupt your life, you should ask your doctor if they might be appropriate.

Progestogen treatment • Progestogens are synthetic versions of the natural hormone progesterone (see pages 44-45), and treatment using them has been advocated on the assumption that premenstrual syndrome might be caused by a progesterone deficiency.

Bromocriptine • This drug is usually prescribed to reduce cyclical breast pain, and some trials have shown it to alleviate other symptoms such as headaches, mood changes and bloatedness.

Oestrogen treatment • This is sometimes used to suppress ovulation when this is the trigger for premenstrual problems.

Contraceptive pill • The combined pill is thought to work for some women because it too suppresses ovulation. However, others find it makes their symptoms worse.

Evening primrose oil (gamolenic acid) • This is effective for breast pain, and some women find it helps with other symptoms too. It is thought that the oil corrects a reduced level of essential fatty acids in the blood of some sufferers.

Mefenamic acid (Ponstan) • This and other anti-inflammatory drugs have been found to improve tiredness, headaches and general aches and pains in some women when taken for five days before menstruation is due to start.

Antidepressants • These may help if premenstrual depression is very severe.

Diuretics • These may be prescribed to correct fluid retention which leads to bloatedness, weight gain and puffiness of the face and fingers.

Many women find that a lifestyle change can be as effective as prescribed drugs. Try following this survival plan.

Premenstrual Syndrome survival plan

Refuse to be a victim • Try to take control of your symptoms. You may not be able to defeat PMS through sheer will-power, but you can try to lessen its impact.

Identify your symptoms • Note any symptoms on a menstrual calender for two months and examine the patterns. You need to be honest: try to sort out what is really there from what you think should be there. Because so many symptoms make up PMS it is easy to assume that every ache or mood-swing is a part of it.

Take control • Once you've identified your symptoms and noted when they cause the most problems, try to plan your life so they cause the least possible disruption. For example, if you know you get bloated three days before your period, cut down on salt which will make it worse. You can brief your family, friends and colleagues about impending mood-swings, make sure you're carrying painkillers to deal with that expected headache and hide the biscuits to help you resist bingeing. You may even be able to organise your work load so as to avoid important meetings and deadlines when you know you will feel low.

Watch your diet • Many women find that what they eat can either aggravate or relieve symptoms. You might find it helps to increase the amount of high fibre foods, pulses, fruit and vegetables and cut down on fats and animal proteins. Some find that caffeine increases their symptoms so you may wish to limit your tea and coffee consumption to two or three cups a day, or switch to decaffeinated. Salty foods will worsen water retention.

Some women find that vitamin supplements containing Vitamin B6, magnesium and Vitamin E help symptoms and that Evening Primrose Oil (0.5-1g daily) is good for breast pain.

Get moving • A couple of exercise sessions a week will help to reduce stress and give you a feeling of well-being. Stretching exercises make you more supple and reduce the stiff back that plagues many women. Even brisk walking will help. Exercise is also a good natural antidote to sleeplessness.

Seek Support   •   Contact the National Association for Premenstrual Syndrome.

What You Need to Know About Your Period

The only normal period is the one that is normal for you. Our periods are as variable as our height, weight and hair colour.

Although it is a received 'fact' that a normal cycle lasts for 28 days, nothing could be further from the truth. Statistical research shows that most women don't have a 28-day cycle, but more women have a cycle of 28 days than any other single length. A recent study of more than 2,000 American women found that the average cycle for 77 per cent was 25 to 31 days in length, but anything between 23 and 32 days is extremely common. It's not uncommon for women to have a regular cycle that lasts for as few as 20 days or as long as 40. About 5 per cent of women have very irregular cycles.

If your periods are consistent, that is roughly the same month after month, then they are normal. A sudden change in your cycle – unusually bad cramps or heavy bleeding, or bleeding that lasts for ten days instead of your usual four may indicate a problem.

In general we lose far less blood than we imagine. The average woman sheds 60ml to 75 ml (between 4 and 5 tablespoons) of blood during a period. Again it is very variable. About 15 per cent of women lose less than 10ml (2 teaspoons) and rarely a woman might lose as much as 120 ml (8 tablespoons). Clinically speaking, a period is 'heavy' when you lose more than 80 ml of blood ($5\frac{1}{2}$ tablespoons). Blood only accounts for a small amount of the fluid lost during your period. About a half to two-thirds of your menstrual discharge is made up of cells from the womb lining mixed up with your normal vaginal secretions.

Your method of contraception can have a major impact on your periods. Women who choose to rely on an intrauterine device (IUD) usually find that their blood flow increases, sometimes by as much as a third. On the other hand, many women using contraception based on the synthetic hormone progestogen (injectable methods, progestogen-only pills and implants – see pages 64-68) find that their periods become irregular and sometimes stop altogether. Other women using these progestogen methods find their blood loss increases.

Strictly speaking, women using the combined pill stop having menstrual periods, instead they have a 'withdrawal bleed' during the seven days each month that they stop taking their pills. This is usually much lighter than a normal period because the womb lining did not receive the earlier signals to plump up. As the womb lining has remained thinner there is less to bleed away.

Period Problems

Painful periods (dysmenorrhoea)

Menstrual cramps are an uncomfortable fact of life for most women, perhaps as many as 70 per cent. They are caused when the uterus contracts to squeeze out the menstrual blood. Sometimes the contractions are so strong that the muscle goes into spasm and temporarily reduces the blood flow to your uterus, causing an oxygen shortage which is experienced as pain. The severity of cramps depends on a number of factors:

Heavier periods • the greater the build-up of womb lining, the greater the womb must contract to slough it away.

Longer cycle   •   many women who have a longer cycle still ovulate at around day 14 of their cycle, which means that just the latter half of the cycle is prolonged. The womb lining has a longer time to build up, leading to a heavier, more painful period.

Sensitivity to   •   prostaglandin is a substance manufactured by the body which promotes
prostaglandin muscular contractions and increases sensitivity to pain. The level of prostaglandin in your blood rises as the level of oestrogen falls, just prior to your period. For reasons which are still unclear, some women's bodies are particularly sensitive to prostaglandin, and they suffer very strong cramps and particularly acute pain as a consequence. In a few women menstrual cramps can be even more intense than that experienced by most women during labour.

If you suffer severe period pains there are several things you can do.

First, if you smoke, give it up! Smoking has a constricting effect on your blood vessels and will make the cramps worse.

Painkillers   •   Painkillers containing aspirin or ibuprofen seem to be more effective than those based on paracetamol. Aspirin helps improve the oxygen flow to your uterus and ibuprofen acts as a muscle relaxant. If the pains are really severe your GP may prescribe an extremely effective painkiller, such as mefenamic acid (Ponstan).

Warmth   •   Warmth can be very comforting, and a hot-water bottle placed across your lower stomach or against your lower back can help to relax muscles.

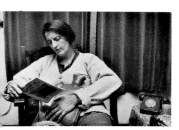

Perhaps the most surprising way of easing the pain is exercise. A brisk walk, jog or work-out may be the last thing you feel like when you are cramping, but it can be an extremely positive way of beating the pain. By working muscles exercise helps to lessen cramping and stimulates the production of your body's natural painkillers, known as endorphins.

Alternatively, some women find relief in yoga, relaxation exercise or massage. Herbal teas made from raspberry leaf and fennel may also be a source of comfort.

Endometriosis

Endometriosis, a condition in which the tissue that usually makes up the lining of the womb begins to grow in other parts of the body, is also linked to painful periods.

Nobody knows quite how the endometrial tissue migrates, but it can cause severe problems as wherever it is situated it responds to the same hormonal signals that are received by the womb lining. It becomes engorged with blood in response to progesterone stimulation and then breaks down ready to bleed away. While our bodies are designed to cope with menstruation (the blood drains through the cervix) there is nowhere for the blood from rogue sites of endometrial tissue to drain. It is trapped and a blood-filled endometrial cyst can form. The bleeding can also result in the formation of scar tissue (adhesions) which can 'glue' the sites of the affected organs together.

The most common sites for the development of endometriotic tissue are around the reproductive organs in the pelvis, and it can often affect the bladder. It can also be found in the stomach, and, more unusually, the lungs and nose. It can even appear in scar tissue such as an old operation wound, as well as in the belly button.

Endometriosis can be painful and distressing. Two out of three sufferers have fertility problems. At the time of their periods many more endure severe pain in the affected area, nausea, pain with urination or bowel movements, diarrhoea and constipation. For women with endometriosis, at any time of the month sex may be painful if there are adhesions in the affected area.

Doctors know little about endometriosis, and there are many theories about why it happens. The most widely accepted explanation is that endometrial tissue is washed back through the fallopian tubes into the peritoneal area where it settles and grows instead of flowing out of the cervix into the vagina. There may also be a hereditary link. You are seven times more likely to develop the condition if your mother or sister suffered from it.

One of the main problems faced by sufferers is that the symptoms, although very painful, can be difficult to diagnose. But if you have pains which worsen just before your period and then decrease and disappear only to start up again a few weeks later, endometriosis should be suspected.

For more information, help and advice about endometriosis, see the addresses at the end of the book.

Heavy periods (menorrhagia)

If the standard 'super' sanitary protection is insufficient to cope with your period or if you frequently leak during the night, it may make sense to seek advice from your GP, especially if heavy periods leave you feeling tired and drained. The blood loss may be affecting your levels of iron and you may have become anaemic and need iron supplements.

Heavy periods can be a sign of various problems.

Fibroids or polyps (non-cancerous growths in the womb lining) are a common cause of heavy bleeding, especially if the blood loss and pain seem to increase by the month. As they grow they increase the surface area of the womb and you lose more blood. These growths are surprisingly common. Probably around a quarter of women have them to some degree, many without realising. Polyps are fleshy, grape-like growths of the womb lining that remain in place when the rest of the womb lining breaks down. Fibroids are growths of fibrous tissue which can develop within the actual womb lining itself (Intramural fibroids) or on the outside of the womb (Subserous fibroids). These are often pain-free in themselves but can grow large enough to press against the bowel or bladder. In some women they grow large enough to create a pot-belly or pregnant appearance. The fibroids commonly responsible for menstrual disturbance are those which grow on the inside of the womb (Submucous fibroids). These sometimes grow on long stalks and extend into the uterine cavity. When this happens, the womb reacts as if it has a foreign body inside it and it contracts especially hard to expel it - hence even stronger cramps.

Fibroids and polyps do not always cause problems and it's quite possible to have them for years without even noticing, especially if they remain quite small. Studies suggest that more than 20 per cent of women over 30 are affected and most are probably quite ignorant of their condition. However, larger fibroids and polyps can hinder fertility as well as causing menstrual problems. If necessary they can be surgically removed.

Heavy periods, particularly ones that last for longer than a week, may be caused by a hormone imbalance such as an oestrogen deficiency. Hormone imbalances are particularly common among young women who are in their early years of fertile life. Sometimes it can take a while for the highly complex monthly cycle to settle down. Doctors can identify if period problems are caused by hormone imbalances by measuring the hormone levels in your blood.

A one-off heavy period, which is also late, may be a very early miscarriage. The bleed is heavy because the endometrium has continued to thicken to support the developing embryo, so naturally when it does break down there is more to lose. Very early miscarriages are extremely common. Nobody knows just how common, as most of them will have been to women who have not even known that they were pregnant.

Lack of periods (amenorrhoea)

Pregnancy is the most common reason for amenorrhoea, and if your periods suddenly stop it is the first thing you should consider if you have had sex since your last period, even if you know you have been scrupulous in your use of contraception.

If pregnancy is not responsible, then one of the following factors may be to blame.

Stress • Anxiety and fear can upset the delicate balance of hormones that control your menstrual cycle. Your periods may suddenly stop because you are under a great deal of pressure at work, or you are coping with a bereavement or other emotional trauma. Once the trauma is over your cycle will return to normal.

Exercise • In rare cases exercise can also switch off the body's reproductive mechanism. This sometimes happens to women who are undergoing gruelling training in the lead up to competition. Both stress and exercise cause the body to produce endorphins (the body's natural painkillers) which can alter the balance of the hormones necessary for ripening of eggs in the ovaries.

Sudden weight loss • In some women a fall in body weight of just 10 per cent can be sufficient to trigger an ovarian shut-down. No one is quite sure how or why this happens. Absence of periods is one of the classic symptoms of anorexia nervosa and yet starving women in the developing countries still retain their fertility. The fact that anorexia is acknowledged to be stress-related has led some specialists to suggest that it is stress rather than weight loss that stops the periods of anorexic women. The matter is still under debate.

Obesity (weighing 20 per cent or more than your recommended body weight) •	If you are extremely overweight your body recognises that it is not in a fit state to bear a pregnancy so it stops preparing itself for a possible pregnancy and it may stop ovulating too. Sometimes weight gain may be a sign of polycystic ovary disease which can cause fertility problems.
Drugs •	Some medications can tamper with the menstrual cycle. Tranquillisers and drugs for high blood pressure, anaemia and some thyroid problems can inhibit menstruation.

In all these cases a woman's periods will return to normal if the cause of the problem is identified and addressed.

Some more unusual reasons for amenorrhea, which are not so easy to address include the following.

Genetic problems •	Some genetic disorders can cause an abnormal menstrual cycle because they affect the reproductive organs. For example, women with Turner's Syndrome are born without ovaries, usually because part of their female sex chromosome is missing. It's an extremely rare condition affecting only one in 3,000 women and, although sufferers may have certain characteristic signs from birth (they're often very short with a broad neck and have webbed fingers or toes), the condition frequently remains undiagnosed until their mid-teens when lack of breast development and absence of periods suggests something is wrong. Women with Turner's Syndrome can often suffer from menopausal symptoms as the rest of us enter puberty.
Radiotherapy or chemotherapy •	This is often used to treat or to combat cancer but can damage the ovaries causing them to age prematurely.
Inflammation of the ovaries •	This is sometimes a side effect of mumps or, much more rarely, a consequence of pelvic tuberculosis which can cause a woman to develop antibodies which destroy her ovaries. This kind of 'inflammation damage'

is difficult for doctors to detect because the mumps doesn't have to be recent. In fact there is evidence to suggest that the damage can be done to the ovaries of a female foetus if her mother has mumps while she is still in the womb.

Premature Menopause   •   The average age of menopause is 50, but one woman in one hundred faces the menopause in her 30s and a small but significant minority of women are hit in their 20s. The causes of very premature menopause are still shrouded in medical mystery. It may simply be that some women have ovaries which are programmed to last ten or fifteen years instead of 35.

When a woman's menstrual cycle stops permanently before the 'normal' menopause it can cause serious emotional and physical problems. Suddenly she has to face up not only to the fact that she may not be able to bear a child, but also to the threat of premature ageing because oestrogen, a hormone produced by the ovaries, maintains skin tone and bone strength.

She will face an increased risk of osteoporosis (brittle bones) because ordinarily the release of oestrogen as part of the monthly cycle helps to build up bone until the time of menopause, when there is a reduction in bone mass. A woman whose ovaries have shut down early faces a reduction in bone mass before she reaches peak thickness (which usually occurs in her mid-30s). For this reason doctors are anxious that women who experience an early menopause should come forward for treatment.

Toxic shock syndrome

Toxic Shock Syndrome (TSS) is an extremely rare condition which can be fatal and some cases have been linked to the use of tampons.

The Syndrome is a rampant reaction by the body to the poisonous effects of a toxin produced by a normally harmless bacterium, 'staphylococcus aureus'. About a third of the population has this bacterium in their gut, nose, armpit or vagina with no ill effects at all. No one knows what provokes the bacterium to go on the rampage and produce the toxin, which is similar to those that cause certain types of food poisoning. But once the toxin is in the blood it can lead to kidney failure, heart damage and death.

If you use a tampon with too great an absorbency, you may increase your risk of TSS by drying out the natural fluids in your vagina which help protect against bacteria.

It is important to get the risk of TSS in perspective. There is less than one tampon-related TSS death each year. This means that if you insert a tampon before driving to work you are far more likely to be killed on the road than to be killed by TSS.

However, you can reduce your risk of TSS even more by:

- using the lowest absorbency tampon you can
- changing tampons at least every six hours
- switching to a towel at night
- always remembering to remove the last tampon at the end of a period.

If you have any of the following symptoms while you are using a tampon, remove it and contact a doctor immediately.

- a sudden high temperature (above 102°F)
- vomiting and/or diarrhoea
- fainting or dizziness
- a severe sore throat.

For more information, help and advice about Toxic Shock Syndrome see the addresses at the end of the book.

				Jan 1	2	3	4	5	6	7	8	9	10	11	12	13	14	15	16	17	18	19	20	21	22	23	
24	25	26	27	28	29	30	31	Feb 1	2	3	4	5	6	7	8	9	10	11	12	13	14	15	16	17	18	19	20
21	22	23	24	25	26	27	28	Mar 1	2	3	4	5	6	7	8	9	10	11	12	13	14	15	16	17	18	19	20
21	22	23	24	25	26	27	28	29	30	31	Apr 1	2	3	4	5	6	7	8	9	10	11	12	13	14	15	16	17
18	19	20	21	22	23	24	25	26	27	28	29	30	May 1	2	3	4	5	6	7	8	9	10	11	12	13	14	15
16	17	18	19	20	21	22	23	24	25	26	27	28	29	30	31	Jun 1	2	3	4	5	6	7	8	9	10	11	12
13	14	15	16	17	18	19	20	21	22	23	24	25	26	27	28	29	30	Jul 1	2	3	4	5	6	7	8	9	10
11	12	13	14	15	16	17	18	19	20	21	22	23	24	25	26	27	28	29	30	31	Aug 1	2	3	4	5	6	7
8	9	10	11	12	13	14	15	16	17	18	19	20	21	22	23	24	25	26	27	28	29	30	31	Sep 1	2	3	4
5	6	7	8	9	10	11	12	13	14	15	16	17	18	19	20	21	22	23	24	25	26	27	28	29	30	Oct 1	2
3	4	5	6	7	8	9	10	11	12	13	14	15	16	17	18	19	20	21	22	23	24	25	26	27	28	29	30
31	Nov 1	2	3	4	5	6	7	8	9	10	11	12	13	14	15	16	17	18	19	20	21	22	23	24	25	26	27
28	29	30	Dec 1	2	3	4	5	6	7	8	9	10	11	12	13	14	15	16	17	18	19	20	21	22	23	24	25
26	27	28	29	30	31																						

Monitoring your menstrual cycle can help you to understand your body. It will allow you to spot patterns that are normal for you and to identify changes.

Photocopy, or re-draw, the calendar above and fill it in using the following symbols:

P – for days when you have your period (you can alter the size of the letter to reflect how heavy the bleeding is e.g. P for heavy days and p for light days)

PMS – for days when you have premenstrual symptoms (or you could use a symbol for specific symptoms e.g. H for headache or C for cramps)

B – for the days you do your breast check

C – for the day you have a cervical smear test

O – for ovulation

Diagram of the menstrual cycle

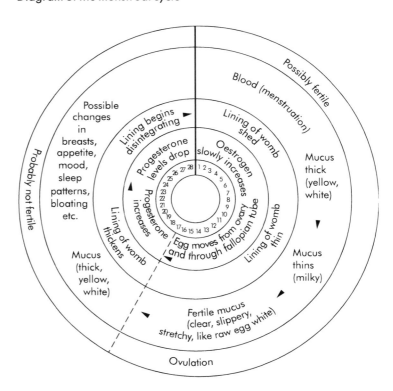

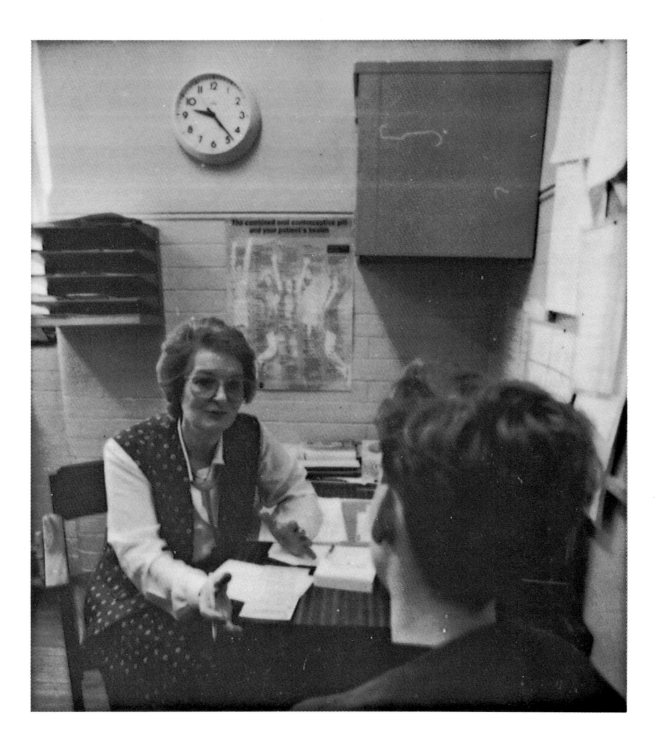

Preventing Pregnancy

Life would be so much easier if we were able to switch our fertility on when we wanted to get pregnant and turn it off again afterwards. Perhaps our granddaughters will be able to do just that. In the mean time our generation has to be constantly on guard against unplanned pregnancy.

The perfect contraceptive would, of course, be 100 per cent effective, safe, reversible, widely available, cheap, convenient and discreet to use, without side effects and beneficial to our health. No such contraceptive exists. Each method is a compromise. Those that best protect against pregnancy (such as the pill or IUD) offer less protection against sexually transmitted infections, while the methods that offer best protection against infections (condoms) are the least discreet. You have to decide what's the most important factor for you. It's a case of 'horses for courses'. Your ideal options when you're in a long-term, mutually monogamous relationship are different from those if you have more than one sexual partner. You have to balance efficacy (see table on page 77) with health benefits, health risks and possible side effects (see below). You have to consider how confident you are about touching your own body, and about discussing your method with your partner.

Ideally we should review our contraceptive options as our lives change. When you're having regular sex with a long-term partner your needs are different from when you're occasionally having sex with someone new.

In reality we seldom review our contraceptive method either because we don't know what's on offer, or because we become stuck in a rut.

This is the latest information on the risks and benefits of all available contraceptive methods. It may help you to decide whether your current method is still the best for you.

Hormonal Methods

The pill

The pill is still the most popular method of contraception in Britain – 48 per cent of women in their early 20s use it, making it more than three times as popular as the condom. Three-quarters of pill users are under 30 – most of them young, single and childless according to the latest statistics. It's also the most popular choice for women who are living with a partner, but not married.

It is likely that pill usage among older women will increase because women are no longer advised to switch to other methods when they reach their mid-30s. Modern pills are safe until a woman reaches her menopause, providing that she is a non-smoker with no health problems.

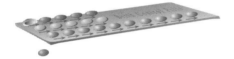

There are two kinds:

The combined pill

How it works • Combined pills contain two synthetic hormones: oestrogen and progestogen. These suppress ovulation so there is no egg for the sperm to fertilise, alter the womb lining and change cervical mucus so as to make it more difficult for sperm to get through.

Health benefits • The pill reduces the risk of cancer of the ovaries and womb lining even long after you stop using it. It regulates the menstrual cycle by reducing blood loss, cramping and pain and may reduce the risk of pelvic inflammatory disease. The pill offers some protection against ectopic (tubal) pregnancy and reduces incidence of benign breast disease by half or more and the risk of ovarian cysts by up to 90 per cent. Other benefits include easing premenstrual symptoms, clearing up acne and reducing the risk of iron deficiency anaemia from heavy periods.

Health risks •   The pill does not protect against cervical cancer or infection by HIV or most sexually transmitted infections. Smoking, high blood pressure, diabetes and high blood fat levels in conjunction with using the pill increases the risks of cardiovascular disease.

Possible side effects •   The pill can cause weight changes (gain or loss), mood changes, spotting between periods, headaches, nausea – particularly in the first three months of use. Side effects can often be resolved by changing to another brand.

It could be for you •   If you are healthy, are not a heavy smoker and have no history of blood clots, heart attacks, strokes, liver problems, breast cancer, high blood pressure, severe headaches or diabetes; if you want a contraceptive that doesn't interfere with sex and are confident that you don't need protection against sexually transmitted infections but need reliable protection against pregnancy.

It's not for you •   If you are a smoker over 35, are very overweight, have abnormal vaginal bleeding, liver or gall bladder problems or are a heavy drinker, have any suspect cancers, suffer from severe depression or are going to have major surgery in the next month, if you or your family has a history of thrombosis or heart disease or if you are liable to forget to take it.

Progestogen-only pill or mini-pill

These pills are mainly used by older women who can't tolerate oestrogen, though almost 6 per cent of women under 40 take it. Doctors are often reluctant to prescribe it because you must take it at the same time each day. If you are so much as three hours out, you lose protection.

How it works •   It causes changes to the cervical mucus and endometrium to make it difficult for the sperm to enter the womb and for the egg to attach itself in the womb if, by chance, it is fertilised. In some women it also suppresses ovulation.

Health benefits • The progestogen-only pill may relieve painful periods and offers some protection against ectopic pregnancy (though less than the combined pill).

Health risks • The progestogen-only pill carries a small risk of ovarian cysts.

Possible side effects • The progestogen-only pill can cause menstrual irregularity (some women stop having periods altogether). Some women suffer weight gain or headaches others report loss of sex-drive.

It could be for you • If you can't use a combined pill because you are a heavy smoker over 35, or if you or your family have a history of heart disease, high blood pressure or thrombosis.

It's not for you • If you have unexplained menstrual irregularities, if you weigh more than 11 stone, if you have had previous ectopic pregnancies or liver disease or you would be unable to remember to take it.

Injectable hormones (Depo-provera or Noristerat)

These are not usually a first choice of contraception because if there are any side-effects they remain until the injection has worn off. Doctors usually recommend 'injectables' if they think a hormonal method is best for you, but you are unable to remember to take the pill regularly. Injections are often recommended for women at opposite ends of the intellectual spectrum – for intellectually challenged women who can't understand the need to take the pill, and for high flyers who are too pressured to remember.

How it works • Injections work in the same way as the progestogen-only pill, but it also always inhibits ovulation. The hormones are injected either every twelve weeks or every eight weeks, depending on the type.

Health benefits • Injections have most of the benefits of combined pills.

Health risks   •   There is a possible connection to osteoporosis or to thrombosis in some women, but there are no proven links with either condition.

Possible side effects   •   Injections can lead to menstrual disturbances – bleeding can be frequent, irregular or absent; weight gain and fluid retention; headaches, changes in mood, depression and sex-drive.

It could be for you   •   If you want to use a hormonal method but can't remember to take the pill; if you have been happy on a progestogen-only pill, but worry about forgetting it; if you are certain you don't want to get pregnant in the next two years or hate having periods (most women stop having them after the second or third injection).

It's not for you   •   If you have any undiagnosed breast lumps, any genital cancers, severe diseases of the arteries or you have had severe side effects on contraceptive pills; if you want to get pregnant in the foreseeable future as it may take up to a year for your fertility to return; if you find irregular periods unacceptable or hate injections!

Implants

Norplant, a system of progestogen implants, is the newest method of contraception to be made available. The same hormone used in the progestogen-only pill and the injectables is contained in six flexible capsules and placed under the skin on the underside of the upper arm. The capsules are effective for up to five years, but can be removed by a trained GP at any time before then, although they are designed to be used as a long-term contraceptive.

How it works   •   The hormone steadily infuses from the capsules into the blood stream. It prevents ovulation in approximately half of the women who use it. In all it thickens the cervical mucus making it difficult for the sperm to penetrate and it makes the endometrium less receptive to any egg that is fertilised.

Health Benefits • These are the same as with the injectables

Health Risks • None known.

Possible side effects • Implants can cause menstrual disturbances. In 80 per cent of users bleeding is frequent, irregular or absent. Weight gain and fluid retention, headaches and changes in mood, depression and sex-drive have also been reported by women using this method.

It could be for you • If you want to use a hormonal method but can't remember to take the pill, particularly if you have been happy on a progestogen-only pill, but worry about forgetting it; if you are certain you don't want to get pregnant in the foreseeable future or are unlikely to be bothered by irregular bleeding.

It's not for you • If you have any undiagnosed breast lumps, any genital cancers, severe diseases of the arteries or you have had severe side effects on contraceptive pills; if you want to get pregnant in the foreseeable future or find irregular periods unacceptable.

Barrier methods

Diaphragm or cervical cap

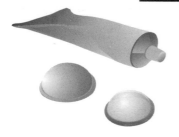

Despite being effective and easy to use, once you've got the hang of it, only a small number of women use the diaphragm. It's most popular among women in their early 30s, but even then only 2 per cent use it. The Family Planning Association thinks their small use may reflect doctors' lack of enthusiasm about fitting them and showing women how to use them.

How it works • A diaphragm is a soft rubber dome which covers the entire cervix (entrance to the womb). A cap works in the same way but is smaller. In the first instance they need to be fitted by a doctor and checked every six months.

Caps or diaphragms must be used with spermicide. They can be put in up to three hours before penetrative intercourse and left in place for at least six hours after.

Health benefits • The diaphragm protects the cervix against human papillomavirus (which is thought to be linked to cervical cancer). Spermicide is known to reduce the risk of gonorrhoea, chlamydia, herpes, trichomoniasis and syphilis.

Health risks • The diaphragm or cap may increase the risk of vaginal infections and augment the risk of urinary tract infections, including cystitis. A tiny number of toxic shock cases in the US have been linked to these methods.

Possible side effects • Spermicide may irritate some women.

It could be for you • If you are happy to delve around in your vagina and can anticipate when you are likely to have sex.

It's not for you • If you find touching your vagina objectionable, are susceptible to vaginal or urinary tract infections or (with the exception of some caps) have very poor muscle tone.

Male and female condoms

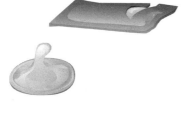
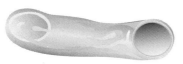

As the female condom has only just hit the market it's too soon to know who's using them. 14 per cent of women under 35 use the male variety. They're more popular with the over 30s who are married with children. Among younger women condom usage appears to increase along with educational qualifications. Women who left school after their GCSEs are less likely to use condoms than those who stayed in full time education.

Condom use is growing. According to the London Rubber Company, which makes Durex, 152 million condoms were sold in 1993.

How they work	•	Female condoms trap sperm by lining the vagina, male condoms do the same by fitting over the penis.
Health benefits	•	Condoms can significantly decrease the risk of contracting HIV infection, herpes, human papillomavirus, gonorrhoea, trichomoniasis, hepatitis B, syphilis and chlamydia and protection is increased if you use a spermicide-coated one. Condoms also appear to decrease the risk of cervical cancer.
Health risks	•	None.
Possible side effects	•	Some people are allergic to latex – if this is the case you could try the female condom which is made from polyurethane, or special anti-allergy male condoms.
It could be for you	•	If you are at risk of sexually transmitted infections (even if you are on the pill) and if you are comfortable about negotiating its use with your partner.
It's not for you	•	If you tend to get too carried away to put it on before sexual contact or if you forget to check you have one before the undressing begins.

Other methods

Intra Uterine Devices (IUDs)

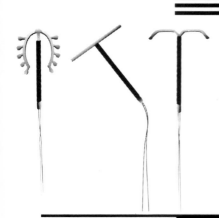

IUDs, sometimes known as 'coils', are mainly used by women in their late 20s and early 30s who are in stable, mutually monogamous relationships. Like diaphragms, many doctors are reluctant to fit them as it is a complicated procedure. IUDs received a lot of bad publicity in the 1980s when they were linked to Pelvic Inflammatory Disease. Modern IUDs are effective and safe, but their dodgy reputation sticks to them which may account for why they are used by just 3 per cent of women under 35.

How it works	•	Mainly by stopping the egg and sperm meeting. It might also stop a fertilised egg from settling in the womb.
Health benefits	•	IUDs may decrease the risk of ectopic pregnancy (this is controversial – some doctors think they increase the risk).
Health risks	•	They may increase the risk of pelvic inflammatory disease if you are prone to sexually transmitted infections. There is also a possibility of infection at the time of insertion.
Possible side effects	•	Some women have more painful, heavier periods and a very few women spontaneously expel the device within the first year.
It could be for you	•	If you are in a mutually monogamous relationship and if you have already had a child, which makes it easier to insert.
It's not for you	•	If you already have painful periods; if you have more than one partner, as this increases your risk of picking up an infection which the IUD would exacerbate.

The sponge

This is used mainly by women who are in stable relationships and are 'spacing births'. Its high failure rate means it is used by very few couples.

How it works	•	The sponge acts partly as a barrier to block the progress of sperm, but mainly as a vehicle for transporting spermicide to the most useful place.
Health benefits	•	It can reduce the risk of gonorrhoea, chlamydia, herpes, trichomoniasis and syphilis.
Health risks	•	May increase incidence of yeast infections like thrush and there is a relatively high risk of pregnancy unless it is used with a condom.

Possible side effects	•	Some women have an allergic reaction to the spermicide.
It could be for you	•	If you are not too worried about the risk of pregnancy and don't mind touching your vagina.
It's not for you	•	If you are significantly at risk of infections or if it would be a disaster if you got pregnant.

Natural family planning methods

These methods are used by less than 1 per cent of women under 35, mainly those who can't use other methods, or don't want to for religious, health or other personal reasons.

They were expected to increase in popularity as a 'green' or 'natural' method, but they have never taken off, probably because of the high failure rate.

How it works	•	You predict, and avoid having sex on, the days when you are most fertile. It is possible to predict your fertile period in a number of ways. If you have a regular cycle you can time it as the fertile time is usually between 12 and 16 days before the start of your period. The most reliable natural method of family planning is the 'sympto-thermal' method which means that you take your temperature every day (it will rise a little just before ovulation) and pay attention to changes in your vaginal fluids (which become wetter and slippery just before ovulation).
Health benefits	•	A greater awareness of what's normal for your body might help you spot any problems, such as infections, earlier.
Health risks	•	None.
Possible side effects	•	None.

It could be for you   •   If you ovulate and menstruate regularly and are conscientious about following your cycle and you don't want to use drugs or devices to prevent pregnancy because of side effects or for personal or religious reasons. You and your partner will need to have an iron will and be prepared to abstain or use a back-up method like a condom or diaphragm during your fertile time of the month.

It's not for you   •   If you are impulsive about when you have sex, are at risk from sexually transmitted infections, object to examining your vaginal fluids, are uncomfortable about discussing sex with your partner or you have an irregular menstrual cycle.

Sterilisation

Sterilisation is mainly used by women who are married, have children and are absolutely certain they don't want any more. 3 per cent of women and 3 per cent of men under the age of 35 have been sterilised for contraceptive reasons.

How it works   •   If the fallopian tubes in the woman, or the vas deferens in the man are cut or blocked, it is impossible for sperm and egg to meet. Although reversal techniques are being developed, sterilisation should always be seen as permanent and irreversible.

Health benefits   •   In women it may reduce risk of pelvic inflammatory disease.

Health risks   •   If pregnancy does occur after female sterilisation there is a higher risk of ectopic pregnancy. There is no protection against sexually transmitted infections.

Possible side effects   •   There are no side effects in women. In men, there may be an increased risk of kidney stones. A man may produce anti-sperm antibodies, but this is only a problem if he contemplates a reversal.

It could be for you   •   If you are certain, beyond all doubt, that you will not want to get pregnant.

The old and the new

Humans have tried to find some way of controlling their fertility ever since they discovered the link between sex and childbirth. As long ago as 3000 BC, Egyptian women inserted pessaries of honey and crocodile dung into their vaginas, Arab women mashed together pomegranates, rock salt and alum to use in the same way. And Aristotle suggested a mixture of frankincense, cedar and olive oil. These bizarre-sounding remedies may well have had some effect since they would have made the vagina more acidic and so hostile to sperm. The principle of the IUD has also been around since biblical times when Arab camel drivers fitted pea-sized stones into the wombs of female camels to prevent them conceiving. Even oral contraceptives have their precursors in early history. An ancient Chinese text recommends swallowing 24 live tadpoles to guarantee five years of freedom from pregnancy. St Albert the Great, patron saint of natural scientists, suggested in the thirteenth century that bees rather than tadpoles should be eaten.

A moistened linen condom first made an appearance in Europe in the sixteenth century, although in Japan men were reputedly using hard sheaths made of tortoiseshell, horn or leather. Casanova used a condom made of sheep gut which he referred to as his 'English overcoat'. Rubber condoms were not developed until the nineteenth century.

The first 'rubber goods' for women, early cervical caps, also made their appearance in the 1800s. They were custom made from a beeswax mould of the woman's cervix. The first modern IUD, a thread pessary, made of silk , was developed by a German doctor in 1909.

Developments in hormonal contraception took off in the 1950s leading to the launch of the contraceptive pill in the early 1960s. Modern pills contain only about one-seventh the amount of hormones of those in the early days.

New methods currently in research include:

Vaginal Rings
- A flexible rubber ring (about the size of a curtain ring) which releases hormones is worn in the vagina. Currently progestogen-only and combined oestrogen/progestogen rings are under development. They will have the advantages of contraceptive pills without the chance that you will forget one. Unlike the current implants you can remove it yourself.

Levonorgestrel IUD
- This method combines an IUD with a slow release progestogen to help control the heavy painful periods suffered by some IUD users.

Monthly injections
- New injections of oestrogen and progestogen are being tested in the hope of finding a way of avoiding the irregular bleeding which is a disadvantage of the current injectables.

Spermicides
- Research continues into new and better spermicides in the hope of finding a product which is effective on its own.

Nasal sprays
- Nasal sprays are already used to shut down the ovaries prior to infertility treatment. Eventually these could be adapted into a method of contraception.

After-sex methods
- Better after-sex, and once-a-month methods are being investigated. They include products which would induce menstruation, block the action of progesterone, prevent implantation or cause the womb to contract.

Electrocution
- A small electrical device has been developed in the US which generates a small current when placed at the top of the vagina. This would immobilise sperm preventing them from passing through the cervix.

Contraceptive vaccines for men and women

- A contraceptive vaccine has already been developed for men, as a precursor to a possible male pill, with promising initial results. Weekly injections of the male hormone testosterone suppress sperm production. The next step is likely to involve implants of testosterone or another sperm-inhibiting hormone.

  Other contraceptive vaccines under research aim to make women produce antibodies to the outer coating of their own eggs. These antibodies would prevent sperm from penetrating and fertilising the egg.

How likely is your contraceptive to fail?

With so many different types of contraceptives on offer, you'd think that unwanted pregnancies would be a thing of the past. Not so!

A report published in the *British Medical Journal* last year showed that the number of unplanned pregnancies was actually increasing. A study of new mothers by Anne Fleissig showed that 31 per cent had had an unplanned pregnancy and 69 per cent had been using a method of birth control at the time of conception.

This seems a good reason to demand better methods, but many contraceptive manufacturers insist that their methods are good and it's we who are at fault for not using them correctly. In the throes of passion it's all too easy to leave caution, and contraceptives, in the bathroom cupboard.

The Family Planning Association has devised two sets of failure rates for contraceptive use.

Careful use

- Careful use estimates how many women will get pregnant if 100 women use the method *precisely according to the instructions* for a year.

Typical use • Typical use estimates how many women will get pregnant if 100 women use the method, 'less carefully', as many of us probably do, for a year.

Method	Careful use	Typical use	Most common mistakes or problems
Combined pill	less than 1	3	woman starts pack late or forgets pill; pill interacts with other medications; woman has diarrhoea or vomiting
Progesterone only pill	1-2	4	woman forgets to take pill at the same time each day
Injections	less than 1	less than 1	woman forgets subsequent injection
IUDs	1	2	woman fails to realise that IUD has been spontaneously expelled
Diaphragm	2	2-15	not enough spermicide; diaphragm not properly placed over cervix; woman doesn't check for holes before use
Sponge	9	up to 25	sponge incorrectly placed over cervix; woman forgets to activate spermicide with water; inherently not effective
Male condom	2	2-15	condom slips off; condom not put on early enough; condom tears
Female condom	insufficient data	insufficient data	
Sterilisation	1-3 per thousand		woman is unknowingly pregnant at time of surgery; tubes spontaneously reopen; careless surgery
Sympto-thermal	2	up to 20	couple fail to abstain or use back-up at the right time

In case of emergency

Contraceptive accidents will happen, but with fast action you can usually prevent pregnancy. Two methods of emergency after-sex contraception are available from doctors, family planning clinics and some hospitals.

Emergency • **Emergency contraceptive pills** (sometimes called morning-after pills or
contraceptive pill   post coital pills) contain similar hormones to those found in combined contraceptive pills, but in a larger amount. However, as they are only taken for a short period of time it is possible for most women to take emergency contraceptive pills even if they are unable, for medical reasons, to take the combined pill.

To be effective, two doses of the pills are taken. The first of these must be taken within 72 hours of unprotected sex, the second 12 hours after the first. The pills either prevent or delay ovulation or prevent a fertilised egg from implanting in the womb, depending on when in the cycle they are taken.

After-sex IUD • **An IUD** can also be used as an after-sex, emergency method of contraception if it is fitted in the five days following unprotected sex. If you choose not to retain it as your contraceptive method it can be removed at your next period.

Both methods of emergency contraception are thought to be very effective. Britain's top contraceptive research clinic, the Margaret Pyke Centre in London, found that just 2.6 per cent of women exposed to pregnancy during the fertile time of their cycle became pregnant after taking the Emergency pill. The IUD failure rate is even lower.

Where to get Contraceptive Help and Advice

You can obtain contraceptive help and advice from any of the following places:

- Your own GP
- A GP other than your regular doctor
- A Family Planning Clinic
- A Brook Advisory Centre (if you are under 24)
- A non-NHS women's health clinic such as those run by Marie Stopes, or the British Pregnancy Advisory Service.

Your local Family Health Service Authority (find the number under 'F' in your phone book) can provide a list of all GPs in your area who offer contraceptive advice – nearly all do – and the details of Family Planning and Brook Advisory Clinics. You can also obtain details of clinics from the Family Planning Association.

Emergency after-sex contraception is available from all the above and from some Accident and Emergency Departments of local hospitals.

All contraceptive advice is completely confidential. Even if your partner is registered with the same doctor as you, he cannot obtain details of what a doctor has discussed with you without your express permission.

A doctor is able to give confidential advice about contraception, and prescribe methods to individuals under the age of 16 as long as:

- he or she believes that the young person is sufficiently mature to understand the consequences of their actions
- he or she has encouraged the young person to confide in their parents
- he or she believes that it will be detrimental to the health of the young person if he or she does not provide contraceptive advice or help.

For help and advice about contraception see addresses at back of book.

Unwanted Pregnancy

Unwanted pregnancy is probably the most common hazard of heterosexual sex.

It is impossible to calculate exactly how many women become pregnant accidentally. Family planning specialists calculate that as many as a third of pregnancies are unplanned. If this is correct then over 300,000 women in the UK face a surprise pregnancy every year.

Not all accidental pregnancies are unwanted – many women are surprised but delighted by an unexpected pregnancy. Others are horrified. Still others are confused and unsure quite what to think. Sometimes the first emotions on the confirmation of an unplanned pregnancy are not the ones that last. Many unplanned and initially unwanted pregnancies turn into much-wanted, much-loved children.

An unwanted accidental pregnancy turns your life upside down – it is a problem you cannot ignore or put off. You may decide to continue with the pregnancy and have a child which you will either raise yourself or place for adoption, or you may wish to end the pregnancy by having an abortion. There is no 'easy' choice.

Regardless of what you decide it is important to discuss the matter with a doctor right away. An abortion is easier to obtain and less traumatic if it is early in the pregnancy and if you want to have your baby your doctor will want to make sure that all is well.

About Abortion

Unlike most of the industrialised countries, Britain does not allow abortion on request at any stage in pregnancy. The Abortion Act, passed in 1967, allows a woman to have an abortion only if two doctors believe that her pregnancy involves a greater risk to her life, to her physical or mental health, or to that of her existing children than if it were terminated. It also allows abortion if the child would be born seriously handicapped.

In practice the law *can* be interpreted liberally. The law allows a doctor to consider 'the actual or reasonably foreseeable environment' of the woman. This means that if a doctor feels a woman would become seriously depressed if she were forced to have the child, the doctor could recommend an abortion for the sake of his or her patient's mental health. Doctors can also take into account the circumstances in which a woman lives. This means that although poverty or bad housing are not directly grounds for abortion, a doctor could decide the stress of having to cope with a pregnancy in such conditions would be damaging to a woman's health.

In 1990, a 24-week time-limit on abortions was introduced except when there is a risk to the woman of 'grave permanent injury' or death. Doctors can also waive the 24-week rule when the foetus is seriously handicapped. However, most late abortions are to women with wanted pregnancies where something has gone tragically wrong either for the woman or the child she is carrying.

It is important to be aware that, even if you clearly meet the criteria of the Abortion Act, a doctor can still refuse to give you abortion advice. The law contains a clause which allows medical staff to refuse to be involved in abortion if it conflicts with their conscience.

In principle, abortion is available on the NHS but there's no legal requirement for any health authority to provide an abortion service. This means that the ease with which you can get an NHS abortion depends entirely on where you live.

As soon as the Abortion Act was passed it became clear the health service was unable to meet women's needs. In response to this charities such as the British Pregnancy Advisory Service (BPAS) and the Pregnancy Advisory Service (PAS) were set up to provide a not-for-profit service for women who were unable to get an abortion within the NHS, but did not have the money to go to a private clinic. These clinics still exist and provide an excellent service.

What happens during an abortion?

Abortion methods change according to how many weeks pregnant you are.

Up to 12 weeks

Between the 8th and 12th weeks of the pregnancy, abortions can be carried out by two methods.

Vacuum aspiration or suction

• The opening in your cervix is stretched from the normal 4mm to the same number of millimetres as there are weeks in the pregnancy. Sometimes a special pessary is placed in your vagina beforehand to 'relax' or soften the cervix. A flexible plastic tube is then passed into the womb and its contents sucked out by an electric pump. The whole procedure usually takes less than two minutes and can be done under a local or general anaesthetic. If a general anaesthetic is given you may need to stay in hospital over night.

After the abortion you can expect some cramping (like severe period pains) for an hour or so, and some slight bleeding lasting for five to ten days.

The 'abortion pill' •

The abortion pill is a relatively new method of abortion. The treatment consists of three tablets of a drug called mifepristone (Mifegyne) taken on one day, and a hormonal pessary inserted two days later. The procedure involves three visits to a clinic: the first to take the tablets, the second (two days later) to have the pessary inserted and the third for a check up, a week after the abortion.

The abortion actually takes place on the second visit, after the pessary has been inserted. The procedure usually takes about six hours during which time you experience quite strong crampy pains.

The abortion pill can only be used in the first nine weeks of pregnancy. It works by blocking the action of the hormone which makes the womb lining hold on to the fertilised egg. Consequently the womb lining breaks down and the embryo is lost in the bleeding that follows. The pessary helps to relax the cervix and speed up the process.

The abortion pill is not suitable if you are a smoker aged over 35.

After 12 weeks

At 12 weeks the foetus becomes too bulky to be sucked away, so abortions are carried out using dilatation and evacuation (D&E) or medical induction. It is usually more difficult to obtain an abortion after 12 weeks of pregnancy.

Dilatation and Evacuation

• You are admitted to hospital the day before the abortion, and given a pessary to relax the cervix. The abortion is then carried out under a light general anaesthetic. The cervix is dilated (as in the suction method) but then the foetus and placenta are removed.

The procedure takes from five to twenty minutes. Recovery is swift, although you may have crampy stomach pains for an hour or so after the operation.

Medical induction

• After 18 weeks D&E procedures become more difficult, and abortions are carried out by inducing labour. Either a prostaglandin pessary is inserted into the vagina every three to six hours, or prostaglandin preparations can be injected into the uterus. An intravenous drip containing a drug used to stimulate labour at full term is often used to make the process more efficient.

Medical inductions can be quite distressing. You have labour pains similar to those experienced when having a baby. Most women are in labour for 11 hours but between 5 and 15 per cent will go beyond 24 hours. The foetus is expelled intact and is nearly always dead.

What about the risks?

Abortion is an extremely safe operation, in fact statistically it is safer to have an abortion in the first nine weeks of a pregnancy, than to carry to term.

Infections are the most common problems with early abortions. One in 20 suction abortions will result in mild infection, one in 50 will lead to an infection requiring hospital treatment. Infections can be treated with antibiotics.

The cervix is torn in one abortion in every 100. If this happens the tear can be repaired with a couple of stitches.

In very rare circumstances the wall of the womb can be perforated by the instruments used in the abortion. This is thought to occur in fewer than one case in every 250 abortions. If this happens abdominal surgery may be needed to repair the wound.

Recent studies show that abortion does not cause infertility, but infertility can be a consequence of blocked fallopian tubes, which can follow an infection. This is why doctors should be scrupulously careful to treat any post-abortion infection.

Most women feel sad and upset after an abortion and most wonder from time to time about what might have happened if they had decided to keep their child. There is, however, no evidence that abortion causes lasting depression or psychological problems.

If you think you're pregnant – and you don't want to be

- Confirm the pregnancy as soon as you can – take a pregnancy test if your period is more than a week late. Modern tests, available over the counter from chemists, cost around £10. Many can tell if you're pregnant the day your period is due, but, as a fifth of all early pregnancies spontaneously miscarry, it's possible to have a positive early test only to find your period starts a couple of days later.

If your period still hasn't started ten days after it's due, make an appointment to see your doctor, family planning centre, or if you are under 24 and there is one where you live, go straight to a Brook Advisory Centre.

It's important to act fast, so insist on an emergency appointment. Doctors calculate the length of your pregnancy from the first day of your last period, so although you're only 'two weeks late', you may be 'six weeks pregnant'.

Your doctor will take another test to confirm the pregnancy, and assess if you meet the legal criteria for an abortion. You are entitled to see *any doctor at any practice for abortion or family planning advice*, so if you feel your own doctor would not be sympathetic, arrange to see someone else. Expect to be asked questions about your medical history, your relationship, and how you feel about the pregnancy.

Your doctor will book you in for a consultation at your local hospital. Often this is when the problems start. Some doctors will phone the hospital to make the appointment there and then but others write, which means a further delay, and it's not uncommon to have to wait another six weeks to see the consultant. If you feel the doctor is unsympathetic and is deliberately stalling you, make an appointment to see another doctor.

If there is a long delay you may have to accept that your only chance of getting an abortion is through a private clinic. Many NHS hospitals simply do not carry out abortions after twelve weeks unless there is a serious threat to your life or physical health. Marie Stopes Clinics, the British Pregnancy Advisory Service (BPAS) and the Pregnancy Advisory Service (PAS) are charitable agencies which provide abortion services at a relatively low cost.

At the hospital the second doctor will confirm that you can go ahead with the abortion, and will arrange a date for you to have the operation.

Abortion services are not obliged to offer post-abortion counselling, but many private clinics and the charity agencies provide it as part of their service.

For general advice about abortion and family planning see the addresses at the end of the book.

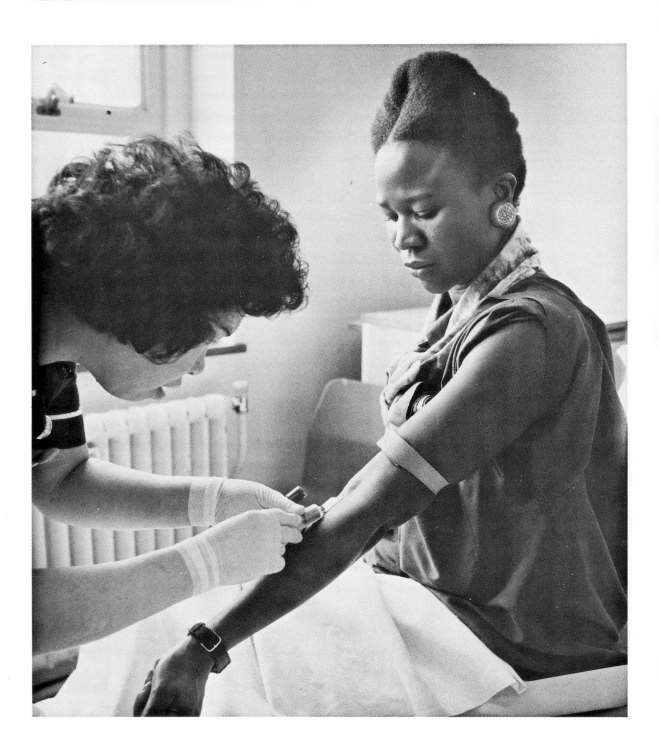

Image and Reality

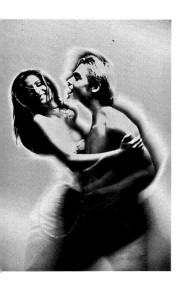

Sex, today, can be a pleasurable, recreational experience. Today's methods of birth control mean that we can enjoy sex without the fear of becoming pregnant and it is accepted that women, as well as men, are sexual beings. Whereas in the past sex was hidden, spoken of in hushed tones and seen as something 'dirty', today it is celebrated. Films, plays, songs and advertising all play on sexual images to get their messages across.

The high profile given to sex can create problems. Usually the images that are flaunted are stereotypes which bear little relationship to reality. Modern films show actors and actresses with sculptured, delectable bodies enjoying a greater variety of positions in one session of sex than many of us enjoy in a lifetime. On the stage and screen sex is nearly always wonderful with both partners enjoying nerve-shattering orgasms.

In real life sex is just simply not like that and it is easy to compare our everyday experience of sex with the celluloid image and feel ugly, boring and inadequate. In real life, however attractive we find our partner, lots of things get in the way of good sex: tiredness, work-worries, the need to do the ironing, fear of waking the children, self-consciousness about our bodies – all these are guaranteed passion killers.

Understanding Sexuality

Sex is extremely important for our sense of individuality. Our self-esteem and sense of well-being are strongly shaped by our view as to whether or not we are sexually attractive to others. Our very personality is often expressed sexually. Our sexual preferences may acquire far greater significance than a description of what we 'do in bed'. Lesbians do not just identify themselves as lesbians when they are having sex with another woman; their sexual preference shapes the rest of their lives too.

Since so much of our personal self-worth rides on sex, it is easy to become anxious, nervous and even scared. The belief that sexual encounters express important statements about individual worth can often intimidate and prevent us from coming to terms with our sexuality. If we regard sexual encounters as tests, it can sometimes be difficult to relax and enjoy the experience.

The starting-point for sexual well-being is to understand its connection with other aspects of our personality. It is simply not possible to experience sexual pleasure on demand. After a hard day's work or a stressful event it is difficult to switch off and feel very sexual. Knowing your sexuality is to know yourself and the problems and pressures you are experiencing. It also works the other way around – the more you know yourself the more you become aware of your sexual needs. Sexual experience and awareness is an endless voyage of self-discovery.

Desire

Is sex merely physical pleasure or is it also about the emotional bonding that comes with intimacy or close relationships? Some people differentiate between what they consider to be purely physical pleasure and a 'meaningful' emotional relationship. Sex is often counterpoised to love and it is often argued that while men are oriented towards physical fulfilment, women are more drawn towards emotional satisfaction. Lust and sex drive are associated with masculinity while romance and sexual passivity are associated with femininity. When these sexual stereotypes are accepted they can lead to all kinds of problems some of which can have very destructive consequences. If a woman feels it's wrong for her to enjoy sex then she may not admit, even to herself, that sex is likely to take place and so she might not be prepared with contraception. If a man feels that he is supposed to know all there is to know he is unlikely to be responsive to his partner's directions. And if people are preoccupied with how they think they ought to behave rather than with what they actually feel there is much scope for misunderstanding.

Communication breakdown

'I really wanted to go out with him again, but I had been brought up to believe that it was 'fast' for a girl to phone a boy – so I didn't call him. Every night I was really upset when he didn't call but I couldn't bring myself to phone him in case he didn't want to see me again. Months later I heard from one of his friends that he had been just as upset that I hadn't called him, but by then it was too late.'

'I knew we both fancied each other, and I had half an idea that we might make love but it seemed really calculating to put my cap in before I went to meet him, and it seemed even worse to take it with me just in case. He might have thought I always carried it in case I met someone I fancied. We ended up having unsafe sex because we couldn't hold back. I worried about it for months.'

'Whenever we've talked about our sexual experience, I've always lied – even though I've never lied to him about anything else. He thinks I've only had about half as many men as I actually have. I know it's stupid, especially as he has had a very promiscuous past, but I'm scared he'll think I'm a slag.'

'I once tried to show him how to touch me, but it was a disaster. He was so insulted. He thought he should know everything about sex, and I should know nothing. Sex was always a disaster, but he thought it was my fault because he said I didn't know how to screw.'

Women can enjoy sex quite as much as men whether it takes place within a permanent or a casual relationship, with someone you love or with someone for whom you simply lust.

However, if you do have casual relationships you need to give careful thought to how you can avoid sexually transmitted infections, including HIV.

Sexual Variety

Our sexual preferences are as different as our taste in food. Just as our favourite dishes change, what attracts us sexually changes too. It is a big mistake to assume that there is a 'normal' or 'standard' sexuality and that other expressions of sexual feelings are 'deviant', 'abnormal' or 'perverse'.

Most people are sexually attracted to someone of the opposite gender (heterosexual) and most people probably want to 'settle down' into a long-term exclusive (monogamous) relationship with a partner whom they love. Most of us have been taught that this is 'normal behaviour', and we may even have grown up believing that it is the only acceptable way of living.

There are, however, a number of alternatives to such a monogamous heterosexual lifestyle.

Homosexual	•	where people are attracted to members of their own gender
Lesbian	•	where women are attracted to other women
Bisexual	•	where people are attracted to members of their own gender as well as their opposite
Celibate	•	where people choose not to share their sexual feelings with another individual
More than one partner	•	at times in their lives some women and men may want to have more than one sexual partner.

Sexual preference is not a fixed thing and it is common and normal for you to find different things desirable at different times in your life.

Knowing Your Body and Desires

Like anything else worth while, the achievement of sexual well-being requires a bit of work. It is worth while to find out how your body works and how it responds to different forms of stimulation. Sex is not merely about genitals. All the senses – sound, smell, sight, and touch – are involved in providing pleasure.

You may find that you feel differently about sex at different times of your monthly cycle. Some studies suggest that sexual interest often peaks at the mid-cycle or just before or during menstruation. There seems to be no obvious reason for this and no reason why you should not enjoy sex at any time during the monthly cycle. Despite traditional reservations regarding sex during menstruation there is no *medical* reason to avoid it, though some cultures forbid penetrative sexual intercourse when the woman is bleeding.

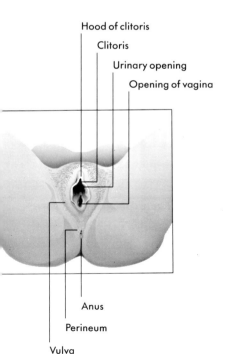

Hood of clitoris

Clitoris

Urinary opening

Opening of vagina

Anus

Perineum

Vulva

Sex is not reducible to penetrative sexual intercourse. Touching, cuddling, stroking, looking and talking can be just as erotic. Certain areas of the body, especially parts of the skin, react with great intensity to touch stimuli. These areas, which are easily sexually aroused, are called *erogenous zones*. Our breasts, nipples, buttocks, lips and the area around the vagina and clitoris make up our erogenous zones. When these areas are touched they spark a physical reaction leading both to local and more general body changes. Physical contact with these areas usually stimulates an increase in the supply of blood which leads to even greater sensitivity. At the same time the body reacts by increasing blood pressure, the pulse rate, breathing and sweating.

The sensitivity of the skin in the erogenous zones is owing to the density of sensory nerve endings that react to touch. The greatest concentration of sensory nerve endings are located around the external genital organs, and the skin around the fingertips, mouth, the areola and nipples. It is in this area that the reaction to touch is most rapid and intense. Within the context of a sexual act the touch stimuli are experienced as sexual arousal.

Other parts of the body, sometimes known as 'secondary' erogenous zones, can also lead to intense physical arousal when they are touched. Parts of the skin which are normally covered, such as the upper part of the leg, especially the inner thigh, are often cited as a particularly sensitive part of the secondary erogenous zones. The neck, eyelids and ears are considered secondary erogenous zones.

The nature and intensity of sexual arousal is not only the direct product of the reaction of sensory nerves. It is shaped by the mind. If you are relaxed and 'in the mood' a touch stimulus is far more likely to turn into a sexual one. If you are tense, bored, tired or just preoccupied, your sexual spark plugs may not fire in the same way. In the last resort our mind is our most vital sex organ. The very same touches which drove you insane with desire on Monday may just be irritating on Wednesday if you're in a different mood.

There are countless books and articles providing tips on the different ways you can enjoy sex. But in the end we all have to work out what we like for ourselves. Just as no one can teach you how to have a conversation, no one can teach you how to have great sex.

Satisfying sex does not always (and for some people it may never) involve a man placing his penis into a woman's vagina. Some people find other ways of touching and stroking far more satisfying. Even if you desire penetration, kissing, licking and stroking can enhance sexual pleasure before, during and after penetrative sex.

Specialist publications provide advice on the different positions and movements for making love. In the end such advice is not a substitute for trial and error. Most women find it most pleasurable to begin with relatively slow and gentle movements. This makes it easier for the two partners to adjust to each other and physically to communicate each other's sexual needs. One of the most pleasurable aspects of penetrative sex can be the slow, deliberate mutually reinforcing movements, where the pleasure gained by one partner enhances that of the other. Most women prefer that during intercourse the two pelvises should rhythmically rub against each other. In this way the clitoris becomes stimulated with every movement.

It is through the stimulation of the clitoris that an orgasm most easily occurs. This can occur during sexual intercourse through a variety of means. During penetration the shaft of the man's penis and/or his pelvis may be used to stimulate the clitoris. Alternatively your partner can stimulate your clitoris by putting a leg between yours, or by stroking your clitoris manually.

Many woman. can enjoy sex without orgasm. Women who have no sensation in the pelvic area owing to disease and injury often find that other parts of their body are readily aroused by sexual stimulation.

Women who rarely or never experience an orgasm may feel anxious, frustrated and even distressed. If you are concerned about this situation, it is useful in the first instance to talk to your partner. Talking can bring to the surface all sorts of anxieties. It can also help establish whether some sort of sexual adjustment in the way the two of you make love is desirable or helpful.

In many cases the difficulty in experiencing an orgasm is connected to anxieties and other underlying personal problems. If talking with your partner does not work then usually sex therapy can help to reduce anxiety. Reducing the level of anxiety helps most women to increase their enjoyment of sexual pleasure. Good coital technique is fine and, with experience, women learn to move in ways which they find most rewarding. But the key to enjoying intercourse is an openness to interacting with your partner. That means encouraging him when he gives pleasure and telling him to change his movements if he does not or if he causes discomfort. Do not keep silent in order to save your partner hurt. Honesty creates mutual trust which weakens the inhibitions which act as a barrier to two people gaining pleasure from each other.

Many people find that their sexual feelings and moods change in the course of a relationship. When you embark on a relationship, everything is new and can be particularly thrilling because of this. After a while you may find that this thrill fades as you become familiar with each other's body. Enjoying sex in different ways, different places and different circumstances may help you to keep the excitement of the unexpected. But familiar sex has its own advantages. As a relationship develops you may find you are more relaxed and less anxious with your partner – this may enable you to explain more readily what you like and what leaves you cold. Just as no two people dance in exactly the same way, so no two people make love in exactly the same way. With a little time you can become expert in each other. Before you can become expert in pleasing and enjoying your partner you need to become expert in pleasing and enjoying yourself. You need to learn how different parts of your body respond to different types of touching. You need to experiment to find what works for you.

Sexual experimentation means trying new things. If something does not work, try something else.

It's Perfectly Normal

Masturbation

Masturbation is an excellent way to learn about your sexual

responses.Freed from the anxiety of having to perform, or the distraction of being worried about another person, we can learn a lot about how we feel and what we like. This teaches us to feel good about ourselves and hence gives us confidence about our sexuality.

Masturbation is often presented as an activity you perform when you haven't got a partner. This is unfortunate because it devalues the importance of self-awareness. It is as valid and as important a form of sexual activity as any other and is a practical way of achieving sexual pleasure. Since masturbation tends to produce the most physically intense orgasms, many women have found this experience as not an inferior substitute but preferable to penetrative sex.

When you feel comfortable with your body, you can teach your partner what you have learnt through exploration of your own body.

Fantasies

Sex and fantasy are inseparable. But fantasies have nothing to do with reality, and there is never any need to feel ashamed or guilty about your imaginings. It is a way we enhance our consciousness of sex. Using our imagination through fantasising is just a cerebral way of arousing our body and enhancing our pleasure of sex.

Most women have a range of fantasies that contributes to their experience of sex. Many women enjoy imagining having sex in strange and unusual places. Other popular fantasises include having sex with a partner in a situation where you risk being caught, watching another couple making love, finding yourself in a situation where you are so desirable that no man can resist you.

The fact that you fantasise something does not mean that you subconsciously want it to happen. It is entirely down to you to decide whether to share your fantasies with your partner. No one can read your mind.

Pornography and erotica

Some women enjoy looking at pornography and find it sexually exciting, others are repelled by it or find it degrading. Only you can decide how you feel about these kind of sexual images.

Sex games

Sex games can be ways of introducing an element of the unexpected into your sex play. Acting out fantasies, dressing up, having sex in new surroundings and using sex toys can be great fun and very exciting. You both need to think carefully about the consequences of your games beforehand and perhaps agree some rules or guidelines. It is important that you both feel comfortable about whatever it is you intend to do, and that you both feel free to call a halt if you feel uncomfortable or distressed.

Different positions

By varying the positions in which you have sex you will find new ways of stimulating yourself and your partner.But remember sexual activity is not a gymnastics competition. No one awards you points for your contortions.

Many couples enjoy oral sex − fellatio (licking and sucking of the penis) and cunnilingus (licking and sucking of the clitoris and vagina). Since oral sex is physically focused on the genitals it can be not only intensely pleasurable but also a little painful. Begin gently and make sure by talking with your partner that you are not licking or sucking too hard.

Anal sex is risky and is illegal between heterosexual couples in Britain.

However, in many women, the skin around and just inside the anus is highly sensitive and anal intercourse can provoke pleasure similar to vaginal intercourse. But the anus was not anatomically constructed for penetration by the penis and it is easy to injure or to infect the anus through penile penetration. To minimise the risks, the penis and the anus must be lubricated with a suitable cream or jelly − one that will not weaken the condom. Never have unprotected anal sex, and under no circumstances should the penis be reinserted into the vagina after anal intercourse. The penis should first be carefully washed to prevent bacteria from infecting the vagina. It should also be remembered that regular anal intercourse can be extremely harmful as it can dilate the anal sphincter to the point where you lose control of its functions.

Celibacy

Despite the importance that we attach to sex, there are times when we are simply not interested in it. Some people either have no sexual desire or alternatively simply do not want to have sex. There is nothing wrong with celibacy. Certainly if you don't want sex, it is important to make it clear to others.

Sex should never take place unwillingly. If at any time you feel that sex is distasteful to you or is a burden just say no and don't feel guilty about it.

Countering Sexual Harassment

Sexual attention is not always welcome and when someone persists it can be demeaning, humiliating and it can undermine your confidence in yourself. Sexual harassment can take place in any situation: at work, at the shops, when you're out for the evening, even at home. Sometimes sexual harassment can be a deliberate attempt to 'put you in your place'. Sometimes it can be a genuine misunderstanding where the person involved does not realise that you find his or her behaviour offensive.

If you are being sexually harassed it is important to make your views about the situation known.

Confronting a harasser

- Try not to lose your temper or shout. Speak clearly and slowly while you look your harasser in the eye.

- Tell the harasser at once that you find his or her behaviour embarrassing/humiliating/ frightening.

- Do not get into a discussion about what the harasser intended. Concentrate on the inappropriate behaviour.

- Do not confuse the message your harasser receives by smiling, laughing or apologising.

- Do not allow the harasser (or anyone else) to dismiss, laugh off or belittle your experience.

- Remember that you are in the right.

- Once you have made your point walk away.

Sometimes it is not possible for us to take control and prevent unwanted sexual attention. Any woman can suffer from rape, sexual abuse or harassment at any time in her life.

Bad sexual experiences can leave emotional scars which affect the way you feel about sex for the rest of your life. If you have endured such a problem, however recent or long ago it was, you can get support and advice from Rape Crisis Centres.

For help and advice about sexual matters see the information at the end of the book

Problem Pains

At some time or another, many women suffer from painful sex. In general, pain on intercourse is called dyspareunia, but pains can have a bewildering variety of causes.

Dryness •
In most cases the pain is caused by lack of sexual arousal. If penetration takes place when a woman is not aroused then the glands that lubricate the vagina are not stimulated and it remains dry. This happens to most women occasionally and a vaginal lubricant is usually sufficient to ease the problem.

Dryness is often caused, around the time of the menopause, by lack of oestrogen. It can be treated with hormone creams, pessaries or HRT.

Infections •
Pain can also be caused by infections such as cystitis and thrush or sexually transmitted diseases such as herpes or gonorrhoea. Penetrative sex should be avoided until the condition has been treated. Pain can also be a symptom of an allergy to a particular spermicide.

Pain on penetration or on deep thrusts can sometimes be a warning of pelvic infections, endometriosis, or even a condition such as a tipped uterus. Consult a doctor if you suffer deep pelvic pain.

Vaginismus •
Occasionally, women suffer from an inability to become aroused or to have penetrative sex. Vaginismus is the involuntary spasmodic contraction of the muscles surrounding the vagina. The contraction of the muscle creates physical pain and helps produce mental stress whenever intercourse is attempted. In such a situation, penetration becomes extremely painful or simply impossible. Vaginismus can be treated by relaxation and dilating techniques. Women suffering from vaginismus are taught to dilate their vaginal muscles so that eventually they can learn to relax them.

Never put up with painful sex. If your doctor refuses to take the problem seriously change to a doctor who is more sympathetic.

For information, help and advice, see the addresses at the end of the book.

Coping with Sexual Infections and Diseases

Many of us still find the very idea of sexually transmitted diseases and infections a major source of embarrassment. There are lots of myths and misconceptions about sexually transmitted problems. In some people's minds they are still associated with poor personal hygiene or promiscuity, and this may make people reluctant to seek help because they are worried that they will face a barrage of disapproval from doctors.

In reality nothing could be further from the case. Infections and diseases which affect the vaginal and vulval area, or the reproductive organs, are simply that – infections and diseases. Just as bacteria may invade your throat or your stomach and cause a problem, so they can invade your vagina or your partner's penis. And just as you may need a course of antibiotics to clear up a throat infection, so you may need treatment to clear up an infection in your vagina or urinary tract. Sexually transmitted infections and diseases are not a punishment for having sex any more than a sore throat is a punishment for talking. If you contract one you have no more cause to be ashamed than if you had caught tonsillitis.

Sexually transmitted infections and diseases do seem to be on the increase, although it is difficult to get firm figures to show exactly how many cases there are each year. The Public Health Laboratory Service collects figures on diseases that are treated at special STD clinics (sometimes called Genito-Urinary Medicine (or GUM) clinics) but it is estimated that 10 per cent of people suffering from these complaints are treated by their doctor. However, the figures, inaccurate as they may be, do show us that many infections are on the rise.

The number of new STD cases rose by 21 per cent between 1981 and 1990 and the number of women seeking treatment was up by nearly 40 per cent compared with a rise of just 2 per cent of men. Most of the increase seems to be owing to a rise in the incidence of herpes, genital warts and chlamydia.

It's an unfortunate fact of life that women are more susceptible to contracting sexually transmitted infections than men. For example, studies show that if a man infected with gonorrhoea has sex with uninfected women he passes on his infection two-thirds of the time. If, however, the infection was the other way round, with an infected woman having sex with uninfected men, she would pass on her infection to one third of them.

Diseases and infections that affect the sexual organs should never be ignored and should always be treated. Many serious diseases have symptoms which are easily mistaken for minor infections, and delays in treatment may allow the problem to take hold, spread into the uterine cavity and cause conditions which can lead to infertility.

Until recently it was thought that the infertility risk from STDs only applied to women. We now know that men's fertility can be affected too. It has been found that infections can interfere with the production of healthy sperm, and problems can remain for long after the infection is treated, sometimes even permanently.

It is important to bear in mind that although the conditions described on the following pages are mainly transmitted though sex, some, like thrush or cystitis, can arise for reasons completely unconnected with sex.

What's normal and what's not

If you are aware of how your body works normally you are much more likely to spot an infection in its early stages.

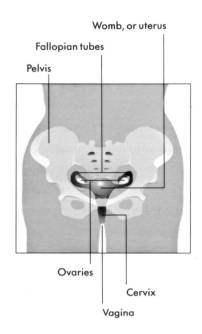

Womb, or uterus
Fallopian tubes
Pelvis
Ovaries
Cervix
Vagina

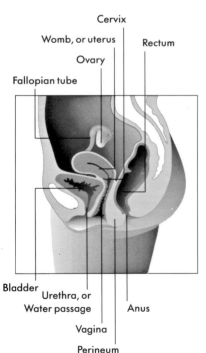

Cervix
Womb, or uterus
Rectum
Ovary
Fallopian tube
Bladder
Urethra, or
Water passage
Vagina
Perineum
Anus

It is normal for all women to have some kind of vaginal discharge – it cleans out the vagina, helps to prevent foreign bacteria from entering the body through this opening and keeps the vagina moist. The fluids are produced by millions of tiny glands in the cervix, the vaginal walls and the introitus (or vaginal entrance). When you are sexually aroused, the glands work in overdrive to lubricate the vagina ready for penetration.

You will probably notice that the amount and consistency of your discharge changes throughout your menstrual cycle. In the first week or so after your period you will probably find that any discharge is scant and hardly noticeable at all. As you approach ovulation (your fertile time of the month) you may notice that your discharge increases in quantity and changes to become very wet, transparent and slippery, like raw egg white. Some women notice that it is also quite stretchy. Most, but not all of this discharge, comes from the cervix which has been stimulated by the rising levels of oestrogen in your blood. The texture and composition of this discharge, sometimes called 'fertile mucus', is sperm-friendly. After ovulation, when progesterone levels climb again, the discharge changes again to become thicker, more jelly-like and white. It may leave a white or yellowish deposit on your pants when it dries.

If you are using a hormonal contraceptive (the pill, implants or injections) you will not notice the same changes throughout the month. Your discharge will remain more scanty and possibly thicker – more like the discharge that other women experience at the beginning and end of their cycles. You will not produce 'fertile mucus'.

If your discharge does not make you sore or itchy and if it does not have an unpleasant smell it is probably normal.

The vagina and introitus is designed to be moist. If this area dries out it becomes itchy, sore and prone to infection. This sometimes happens as you approach menopause and the hormone levels in your body change.

You may want to ask a doctor or pharmacist to recommend a special lubricating gel or hormone cream.

In their normal state, your vaginal secretions have a slightly acid pH balance. This acidity is maintained by 'friendly' bacteria, and if their number is disturbed then the finely tuned balance can be upset allowing possible invasion by 'hostile' unwanted bacteria and yeasts. Unless your doctor or a pharmacist thinks you have a problem which will be eased by the use of a particular lubricant, wash or other special product, it is best to avoid using special washes, wipes and vaginal deodorants unless you have a specific problem. Over-zealous cleansing and use of vaginal douches, wipes and deodorants can sometimes upset this natural balance and make you more prone to infections.

If you have a normal discharge you should allow your body to take care of itself. Simply wash your outer vaginal area with a gentle soap twice a day. Never try to cleanse inside the vagina. Never try to mask a pungent or unpleasant smell with deodorants – it may be an infection which needs treatment.

Prevention is better than cure

If you are having sex with someone who you think may suffer from an infection it makes sense to practise 'safer sex' – activities which do not involve an exchange of body fluids.

You can reduce your risk of most sexually transmitted infections and diseases by using a condom when you have penetrative sex. If you need to use an extra lubricant it is very important that you use a water-based lubricant such as KY jelly. Oil-based lubricants such as Vaseline or baby oil damage the rubber. Massage oils and some sun oils and creams can have this affect too. So take extra care if you use them before you have sex. The spermicide Nonoxynol-9 is also thought to kill the HIV virus. The lubricants on some condoms already contain it, but you may wish to use it anyway to give you extra protection. Nonoxynol-9 causes irritation in some people and if you feel sore or itchy after using it you should switch to another spermicide.

Possible signs of an infection

You should seek the advice of your GP or a doctor at a special clinic if you develop any of the following symptoms.

1. An unusual change in the amount or type of moisture in your vagina. It is usual for the secretions to change throughout the month, but you should seek advice if:

    - there is more discharge than you would normally expect
    - it looks different, especially if the colour is unusual
    - it feels different
    - it has a strong, unpleasant or unfamiliar smell
    - it makes your vagina itch or feel sore or irritated.

2. Sores, warts or blisters near the vagina or anus.

3. A rash or irritation around the vagina or anus.

4. Pain or burning when you pass urine, or the desire to pass water more frequently than usual.

5. Pain or discomfort on intercourse.

You should seek medical advice, and get your partner to seek advice, if he develops any of the following:

- a discharge from his penis

- Sores, warts or blisters on or near the penis or anus
- a rash or irritation around the penis or anus
- pain or burning when he passes water, or the desire to pass water more frequently than usual
- pain or discomfort on intercourse.

Sexual infections and how they are treated

It is a strange fact that the sexual infections that nearly everyone has heard of are the life-threatening but uncommon ones. The most common, like chlamydia, are seldom discussed. In the following pages we have outlined what the various infections and diseases are and how they are transmitted and treated. The star rating gives you an idea of how common each problem is and how much of a threat to your long-term health it poses.

It is important to remember that even if something poses little long-term risk to your health and fertility, it may still cause intense pain and discomfort and no good doctor will feel that it is a waste of time to treat you for it.

Long-term risk factor: • The greater the number of stars, the greater the threat to your health

Incidence: • The greater the number of stars, the more common the infection

HIV/AIDS

Long-term risk factor: *****
Incidence: *

Once HIV gets into the blood stream it damages the body's immune system by interfering with the very cells which protect us against infections and diseases. Eventually most people who have been infected with HIV will develop Acquired Immune Deficiency Syndrome (AIDS) although this may take very many years. About half of those known to be infected with HIV develop AIDS within ten years. AIDS is diagnosed when the immune system of the sufferer is no longer able to fight and various 'opportunist' infections and diseases take hold.

HIV can be transmitted by sexual intercourse as well as through infected blood entering your bloodstream (perhaps by sharing drug injecting equipment or by transfusions with infected blood).[1] It can also be transmitted from a mother to her child during pregnancy or through her breast milk.

Someone who is infected with HIV can remain free from symptoms for many years while still being infectious. It is possible to identify if someone is infected by examining their blood for antibodies to the virus. However, since it can take the body up to three months to build up these antibodies the test cannot confirm if you have contracted the virus in the last twelve weeks.

Although there are articles in the newspapers about AIDS almost every week it is still a very rare disease.HIV is still rare too. But because it is deadly and there is no cure it is important to protect yourself against it.

Should I have an HIV test?

A blood test will tell you whether or not you have been infected with the HIV virus. It works by detecting antibodies that your body makes when it is invaded by the virus.

A negative result means that your body has not produced antibodies to HIV because you have probably not been infected by the virus. However, it can take as long as three months (and occasionally longer) from the time of infection for the antibodies to show up in tests. So it would show whether you were infected by a man you had sex with six months ago, but not a man you had sex with last week. However, if you suspect you may have been infected recently you should still seek medical advice – even before the test can confirm whether your suspicions are justified.

   [1] All blood used in the UK has been screened to ensure it is free from infection.

A positive result means that HIV antibodies have been found in your blood, and that infection with HIV has occurred. (This may not be so for babies of infected mothers who test positive because antibody tests on new born babies reflect their mother's HIV antibody status.)

A positive HIV test does not mean you have AIDS, but it does mean that you are infectious and can pass on the virus to other people.

Your doctor can arrange for you to have an HIV test or you can have one at a GUM clinic.

If you decide to have the test

It is important to talk to a health advisor, counsellor or doctor before you have an HIV test, to consider how the knowledge might affect you. The result, and the fact that you have been tested, is confidential between you and your doctor and other staff involved in your care. Your doctor cannot inform your employer, or other members of your family even if they are patients at the same clinic or surgery.

Only *you* can decide whether it is right for you to have the test. You might want to consider these points:

- Treatments which may slow the progress of HIV infection and delay the onset of AIDS are available. If you know you are infected you could take advantage of these.
- Knowledge that you are infected may help you to make important decisions about your job, your sex life and whether or not to have a family.

On the other hand:
- If you are infected you may have difficulty getting life insurance or a mortgage. Even if the test is negative insurance companies ask questions about your lifestyle which could lead to a higher premium.

• Being HIV positive unfortunately still carries a stigma and, if you tell people, you may have difficulties with your family and friends or even your employment and housing.

Before you decide, you might like to ask yourself:

• Am I likely to be infected?
• Do I need the result to help me make an important decision?
• Who would I tell about the result?
• How would the result affect my housing or employment?

See addresses at back of book for advice.

Hepatitis B

Long-term risk factor: ****
Incidence: **

The Hepatitis B virus is highly infectious and can be transmitted through body fluids such as semen and vaginal secretions and through blood. Usually it is contracted through sex or contact with drug injecting equipment.

Although our awareness of HIV is far higher than that of Hepatitis B, the latter is far more infectious. It has been estimated that at least 0.1 ml of blood (about two drops) is needed to transmit HIV while Hepatitis B can be transmitted by just 0.00004ml (a tiny fraction of one drop). This means that doctors, nurses and other medical personnel who handle injecting equipment are at particular risk. Because Hepatitis B is so infectious it can be passed on through sharing a toothbrush or razor or even 'wet' kissing if there are any tiny traces of blood in the saliva. Unlike HIV, the virus can also survive in dried blood for up to a week which means that the surfaces of razors and surgical instruments can remain infectious that long.

Symptoms of Hepatitis B infection can take up to six months to develop. They range from flu-like aches and pains and tiredness to the yellowness of skin and eyes that is associated with jaundice. Some infected people never develop symptoms although they remain carriers of the disease and are able to infect others. Doctors can easily identify the presence of infection, whether symptoms are present or not, by a blood test.

Even in carriers who remain free from symptoms, Hepatitis B can lead to progressive liver damage and even liver cancer as a result of the continued infection.

The virus is far easier to prevent than to treat as a vaccine has been designed to give immunity. There is no effective medical cure for acute Hepatitis B infection but for those who are carriers treatment is available using injections of 'interferons' to boost the body's natural defence. The injections are thought to offer about a 25 per cent chance of combatting the virus.

Genital herpes

Long-term risk factor: ******
Frequency: *******

Genital herpes is caused by the Herpes Simplex Virus (HSV) which tends to affect those parts of the body where two different types of skin meet, for example, the angle of the mouth, the genital area, the skin around the anus and more rarely the eye.

There are two types of Herpes Simplex Virus: type I and type II – either can infect the parts of the body mentioned above but in general HSV II is more likely to be responsible for genital herpes, whereas HSV I is more likely to infect the face.

There is no cure for herpes. Once you are infected by the virus you have it for life. However, that does not mean that it is a constant problem.

The first herpes attack is usually more severe than subsequent attacks, should they occur, because during the first attack you begin to build up antibodies to the virus. Many sufferers are lucky and only have one attack. The symptoms are easily recognisable compared with some other

STDs. First you usually feel a burning or tingling sensation on the area around your vagina. This is followed by itching, and a crop of small blisters which turn into red excruciatingly painful ulcers. These rapidly crust and turn into sores which take from seven days to two or three weeks to heal. During the time that the blisters are present and for around five days afterwards, you are infectious and can easily pass the virus on to anyone who you have sex with. When you are free from symptoms you are not infectious. A first attack can also be accompanied by fever and pain and swelling in the groin. Occasionally this can be bad enough to necessitate admittance to hospital.

Many people find that after the initial herpes attack, recurrences are triggered when they are suffering from stress and it's not uncommon for women to find that attacks are linked to their periods.

An anti-viral drug called acyclovir (Zovirax) has recently been developed and it is effective at controlling symptoms. It can either be applied as a cream or, in severe cases, taken as tablets. Some women find that they get pain relief by applying ice compresses and bathing the sore areas in a solution of one teaspoon of salt to a pint of water.

It is important to remember that a condom will not protect against herpes infection unless it is able cover all the blisters, and also that unlike many STDs, herpes can be transmitted through non-penetrative sex if areas on the outside of the genitals are affected.

Genital warts

Long-term risk factor: **

Frequency: ***

Genital warts, like warts on your hands or feet, are caused by a virus. They can be transmitted sexually or they can just grow in the genital area much as they grow on other parts of your body. In women, genital warts may be difficult to spot if they grow inside your vagina. They can be as tiny as pin heads or take on a distinctly 'warty' cauliflower appearance. The virus has a long incubation period and warts may not appear until six months after you have been infected.

There are several strains of the wart virus. Some have been linked to the changes in cervical cells which can lead to cancer. Thus it is extremely important for any woman who has either suffered from genital warts herself, or has had unprotected sex with a man with genital warts, to have a smear test. If the wart virus is found on the cervix she will need yearly smear tests.

Warts on the external genital area can be treated with a special liquid which dries them up in about a week. Warts in the vagina are usually treated by freezing or by laser.

Condoms will only protect against the wart virus if they cover all the affected areas. As with herpes, genital warts can be transmitted through non-penetrative sex, if areas on the outside of the genitals are affected. Condoms and diaphragms can, however, protect the cervix.

Syphilis

Long-term risk factor: *********
(if untreated)
*
(if treated)

Frequency: *****

Syphilis is a very serious condition, and is often hard to detect in women. In men the first sign is usually a painless, but clearly visible, ulcer on the penis or anus which appears two weeks after infection. In women the same kind of ulcers usually appear on or near the vagina or anus, but they are far more difficult to detect and may go undetected. Some women become aware that something is wrong because their labia (vaginal lips) become swollen and tender. The most obvious sign of infection may be a faint pink, spotty rash on the chest, back and arms which persists for several weeks. It can be identified through a blood test.

Syphilis carries two dangers for a woman if untreated. The most immediate danger is that if she becomes pregnant her child will become affected while still in the womb. The more long-term danger is damage to the nervous system which can lead to insanity and, in some instances, death.

The disease is completely curable if treated in its early stages with high doses of antibiotics.

Chlamydia

Long-term risk factor: **

Frequency: ****

Chlamydia is the single most common bacterial sexually transmitted disease. Although it is often symptomless, left untreated it can cause severe damage to your fertility. Chlamydia is thought to be responsible for up to 70 per cent of pelvic inflammatory disease (see pages 118-119) and it can spread into the fallopian tubes causing damage and scarring. Chlamydia during pregnancy can lead to an increase in ectopic pregnancy, premature birth or even stillbirth. There is also the possibility that it can lead to eye infections and pneumonia in the newborn baby.

Around one woman in ten is thought to carry the infection, most without knowing it.

In women, chlamydia can be symptomless, although sometimes there is a slight increase in vaginal discharge or a vaginal irritation or burning sensation on passing water. In men the disease is more obvious and usually causes a burning pain on passing water and sometimes a white discharge from the penis.

Once diagnosed, usually through taking a vaginal swab, chlamydia can be treated with antibiotics. You should ask for a test if you have any of the above symptoms or any pelvic pain. If you have a number of sexual partners it is wise to have occasional checks at a clinic. Using a condom will provide protection against infection.

Trichomoniasis

Long-term risk factor:

Frequency: ***

Trichomoniasis is caused by a tiny single cell parasite which causes an infection in the vagina and urethra. It is usually sexually transmitted, but the organism can survive at room temperature on moist objects, so it is theoretically possible (although unlikely) that it could be passed on by a shared towel or sponge.

In men it causes a yellowish-green thin discharge from the end of the penis, and pain when passing water. Sometimes men can experience no symptoms at all but can still be infectious.

In women, although it can be symptomless, it often causes a yellowish-green thin vaginal discharge which can have a slightly frothy appearance. The discharge often has a strong, rather fishy odour which becomes particularly strong after sex without a condom.

Trichomoniasis is treated with a short course of antibiotics, usually metronidazole (Flagyl).

There are no long-term health implications for the disease, although some doctors think it may encourage the development of genital warts. Untreated trichomoniasis may clear up after about three weeks but you should still be checked by a doctor for other infections as nearly one woman in every five with trichomoniasis also has gonorrhoea.

Gonorrhoea

Long term risk factor: ***
Frequency: ***

Gonorrhoea is the second most common sexually transmitted bacterial disease in women. Left untreated it can spread and cause pelvic inflammatory disease (see pages 118-119).

The main symptom in women is a copious vaginal discharge which may be thin and watery and possibly yellow or green in colour.

In men, it causes a yellow or white discharge from the end of the penis and pain or discomfort when passing water. Sometimes there can also be an irritation or discharge from the anus. The symptoms usually start within three to five days of infection, and may be accompanied by 'fluey' aches and pains. These symptoms may last for around ten days, then it may appear to clear up, while the sufferer remains infectious.

Gonorrhoea may be difficult to spot as it has been estimated that fewer than a third of infected women suffer this noticeable discharge.

This can cause major problems. Symptomless women sufferers are not only infectious, they may also be in danger of damaging their long-term fertility. Occasionally the bacteria pass up into the fallopian tubes where they can cause infections which in turn may lead to scarring or blockages.

Once diagnosed, gonorrhoea can be treated with antibiotics. Using a condom will lower your risk of contracting, or passing on, the disease.

Bacterial vaginosis (BV)

Long-term risk factor:

Frequency: ****

BV is often mistaken for thrush as it can cause vaginal irritation, but the symptoms are quite different. A woman with BV usually notices a whitish-grey thin discharge with a strong fishy smell, sometimes so pungent it can be smelled through clothes.

The infection is caused by the bacterium, gardnerella, which interacts with anaerobic bacteria. It usually occurs when the acidic balance of the vagina is altered, especially if you are using an antibiotic. In some women the slight change in acidity that occurs with contraceptive pill use, or even the change that occurs naturally just before a period, is likely to spark an attack.

Once you have had it a first time, BV has a very high recurrence rate, which is not necessarily linked to sex, although sex can be a trigger if the problem bacteria are introduced into your vagina during it.

Antibiotic treatment is extremely effective, and should be taken by both partners. If you find that you are prone to recurrences you may find it helpful to bathe your vagina in a mild vinegar and water solution. However, it is important to have BV properly diagnosed in case you have wrongly identified the symptoms and you really have gonorrhoea.

Thrush

Long-term risk factor:
Frequency: *****

Thrush is the most common cause of 'vaginal itch'. In a recent survey of more than 4,000 women aged between 16 and 60, 45 per cent said they had had at least one attack. Unfortunately more than a third of sufferers have attacks at least once a year.

Thrush is caused by a yeast-like fungus, candida albicans, which burrows into the cells which line the vagina. Most people have a certain amount of candida in their intestines, and many women have it constantly in their vagina without any problem at all. Normally the vaginal secretions are too acidic to allow the fungus to take hold, and additionally it is kept in check by other bacteria naturally present there. However, if the vagina's acidity falls, thrush can overrun it causing an infection.

The symptoms are a thick, white 'curdy' discharge. The vagina may feel sore and extremely itchy and it may be painful to urinate.

Men can suffer from thrush too, the symptoms being itching and redness on the penis – usually on the glans.

Thrush is effectively treated with anti-fungal creams and pessaries which are now available from pharmacies as well as on prescription. Some women find that live natural yoghurt, inserted in the vagina using a tampon, or bathing the vaginal area in a solution of vinegar and water, is sufficient to cure a mild attack. However, if symptoms persist for longer than a week despite treatment it is important to see a GP to confirm that you have correctly diagnosed your condition and not mistaken one of the other vaginal infections for thrush.

Avoid nylon pants, tights and tight trousers if you are prone to thrush as they create the warm moist conditions that thrush likes best. Some women find that they are particularly susceptible to attacks when they are under stress. It is also particularly common during pregnancy.

Cystitis

Long-term risk factor:

Frequency: *****

Cystitis is the most common urinary tract infection in women. It can be caused by a reaction to 'foreign' bacteria, which normally live happily in another part of the body, finding their way into the bladder. But it can also be a by-product of other vaginal infections or caused by friction to the urethra by tight clothes, or bruising, perhaps during vigorous sex (often known as honeymoon cystitis). Some women even suffer cystitis as an allergic reaction to perfumed bath products, or to something they have eaten. Many women are prone to it when they are under stress and allow themselves to become run down. Frequent cystitis attacks can also occur as an unpleasant consequence of the menopause.

Cystitis is usually experienced as the need to urinate frequently – even when there seems to be no urine to pass. This feeling is usually accompanied by a burning pain often described as being like 'peeing razor blades'. The urine may be cloudy or even tinged with blood. Back or abdominal pain is common and some sufferers may run a temperature. Men can suffer from cystitis too, but they generally have a lower incidence of infection than women. They should always seek medical advice if they have these symtoms.

The infection can be treated with antibiotics, and medical advice must be sought if the attack lasts for longer than two days, or if there is blood in the urine. Left untreated, persistent cystitis can spread to the kidneys and cause serious inflammation.

Self-treatment is often very effective. Many women find they can abort an attack by taking action as soon as the symptoms start. The best course of action is, at the first twinge, to drink a pint of water to dilute the urine. Every hour, for the next three hours, drink a solution of a quarter pint of water into which a teaspoon of bicarbonate of soda has been dissolved (check with your doctor first if you have high blood pressure or heart trouble). This reduces the acidity of the urine which slows down the rate at which the bacteria multiply. Drink at least a pint of liquid every twenty minutes to keep you urinating. After the first few trips to the loo the pain should begin to subside.

Collect a mid-stream sample of your urine in a sterile (boiled) jar as soon as the attack starts. Take this to your doctor who can test it to see if you need antibiotics.

Pubic lice

Long-term risk factor:
Frequency: ******

Pubic lice are sometimes called crabs because that is exactly what they look like. The louse (phthirius pubis) is a tiny, yellowish-grey parasite, about a millimetre long, with three pairs of claws and four pairs of legs. They live in the pubic area, moving by swinging from hair to hair and feeding by sucking blood through the skin. Each louse lives for just 30 days but during her lifespan each female lays around three white eggs (nits) a day which are attached to the pubic hairs.

Lice can be treated with special lotions and shampoos obtainable from pharmacies. After treatment clothing and bedding should be washed and mattresses treated to prevent reinfestation.

They can be picked up by close body contact – and not necessarily sex. You can just as easily pick them up from unclean sheets or from borrowed clothes.

Pelvic inflammatory disease

Long-term risk factor: ****
Frequency: **

Pelvic inflammatory disease (PID) can range from a mild, virtually symptomless condition to an extremely serious, occasionally life-threatening disorder.

There is still a great deal that doctors do not know about PID, however there is now agreement that it is a bacterial infection and that usually the organisms responsible have entered the body through the vagina and worked their way up through the cervix into the pelvic cavity. The bacteria responsible for gonorrhoea and chlamydia are thought to be the worst culprits, although other bacteria, particularly some that normally exist harmlessly in the bowel or the gut, are believed to play a part too.

It is thought that sometimes the rogue bacteria may be introduced into the pelvic cavity when the cervix is dilated (opened) during childbirth or miscarriage, an abortion – or even during the fitting of an intrauterine device (IUD). It is now regarded as 'good practice' for a doctor to screen women for vaginal infections, particularly chlamydia, before fitting an IUD or carrying out an abortion. Some doctors even prescribe women a prophylactic ('just-in-case') course of antibiotics, although other doctors argue that antibiotics are already overused and should not be given unless absolutely necessary.

PID is difficult to diagnose, because its symptoms can differ greatly between women. It may make its presence felt as an acute (sudden, severe) infection or a chronic (long-term, lower-grade) infection. In its acute form, the abdominal pain can be so severe that it is possible for doctors to mistake it for appendicitis.

Once acute PID has been diagnosed it is treated with antibiotics. In very severe cases a woman may need to be admitted to hospital so that drugs can be given intravenously. Bed rest is often recommended as any vigorous activity can increase the inflammation and slow down healing. It can be as long as three or four weeks before a woman is back on her feet.

In some ways chronic PID is just as difficult to deal with as the infection may have been present for many months before it is identified. Symptoms may include constant abdominal pain or discomfort, weakness, tiredness, and very heavy painful periods. In a mild case there may be no noticeable symptoms. However, even an almost symptomless attack of PID can cause infertility by permanently scarring the fallopian tubes through which eggs must pass if they are to be fertilised.

Scarred fallopian tubes significantly increase the risk of an ectopic pregnancy if fertilisation does occur, and it has been estimated that women who have suffered from PID have a sevenfold risk of ectopic pregnancy. In addition, the presence of scar tissue may increase the risk of recurrent infection and it can cause pain during sex.

Early treatment lessens the risk of all these problems. This means that if you start to experience any persistent pelvic pain or discomfort (other than your normal amount of menstrual discomfort) you must seek medical advice.

Where to Go for Help

If you think you might have caught an infection, whether you have symptoms or not, go to either a clinic that specialises in genito-urinary infections or to your GP.

You may find your problem will be identified and treated more quickly if you go to a clinic. Clinics are able to process the results of tests immediately and issue you with any drugs you need there and then. Your doctor will probably have to send samples off for analysis and when he or she gets the results they may have to refer you to a clinic anyway.

Clinics exist to treat people of all ages – no matter how young or old you are. For some you will need to make an appointment, but in many clinics you are simply able to walk in. It is a good idea to phone up and find out whether or not an appointment system operates.

How to find your nearest clinic

Depending on where you live, the clinic might be called a

- genito-urinary medicine (GUM) clinic
- sexually transmitted disease (STD) clinic
- special clinic
- special treatment centre

For the address, look in the phone book under genito-urinary medicine, STD or VD, or phone your local hospital or Family Health Services Authority (FHSA).

What happens at the clinic?

The staff at the clinic are trained to treat sexual infections efficiently and confidentially. They will not pass information about you to anyone, nevertheless some people prefer to give a false name. This is not really necessary, but if you feel more at ease doing it, make sure you give a name you will remember!

When you see the doctor you will be asked to describe any symptoms you have had and about your general health. You will be asked when you last had a period, so try to remember the date before you see the doctor. You will also be asked quite a lot of intimate questions about sex, including whether you have a regular partner, and if you have had sex with anyone other than your partner. You may be asked about the kinds of sex you have had recently, for example whether you have had oral sex.

Try not to be too embarrassed and remember that the doctor spends all day every day talking to people about these things so he or she is unlikely to be shocked by anything you say. Always be honest. The doctor asks questions to enable her to diagnose your problem. Tell the doctor if you are pregnant, because some treatments may affect the foetus in the womb.

After the initial discussion you will be given a thorough check up. You will probably have to provide a specimen of urine and have some blood taken (for a routine syphilis test). Your blood will not be tested for HIV unless you have asked for this to be done. The doctor will examine your genital area and also examine the inside of your vagina, taking some samples of your vaginal fluids as she does so. This is very similar to having a routine smear test. It is not painful but it may be uncomfortable.

If you feel uneasy about being examined by a male doctor, ask if you can be seen by a female doctor or if a female nurse can stay with you while you are examined.

Sometimes the doctor will be able to tell you immediately which infection you have and will issue you with a prescription or the necessary treatment there and then. Otherwise you may be asked to return a few days later for your test results.

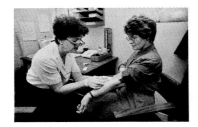

If you are given a course of medicine, you must complete it – even if the symptoms go away in just a few days. If you abandon a course of antibiotics before you finish it it is possible that the infection could remain and may even develop a resistance to treatment.

A visit to a GUM clinic

'I felt really embarrassed about going. I thought I might see someone there I knew – although that was a really dumb worry because it meant that they would have something wrong too.

I didn't have to make an appointment, but when I phoned the receptionist said that people were seen in the order they arrived and as the clinic was really busy, you could wait hours. I wanted to get in and out really fast so I turned up at 9 a.m. even though it didn't open until 10 a.m. I couldn't believe it but I wasn't the first.

There were two waiting areas: one for men and one for women. I was glad, but I could see it would be a problem if you had come as a couple. The worst thing was that there was nothing to read except ancient copies of Hello! If ever you have to go to a special clinic, take your own book.

When you arrived you were given a form to fill in with your name, date of birth, contact address, etc. Then you were allocated a number. This was a really good idea because it means your anonymity is protected. When it was my turn to go in the nurse just called my number. I was really relieved because my name isn't a very common one.

The doctor was nice but a bit brusque and I found it difficult to answer his questions honestly. You always want to say what you think you should say rather than the truth. It was especially difficult when he asked me if I had had sex with anyone other than my husband in the last year – because I had, but nobody knew about it. In the end I was straight about it because the doctor explained that no one would tell anyone anything out of my notes.

I was nervous about the examination. First I had to go into the toilet and produce a sample of urine. It's really hard because the jar you have to pee into is quite narrow. The nurse then showed me into a small room and took some blood from my arm. Then I had to take my jeans and pants off and lie on a trolley. When the doctor came in he asked me to put my feet up on some Y-shaped sticks and he shone a bright lamp up between my legs. He slid the speculum into me just like they do when you have a smear test. It didn't hurt at all, but it felt very cold. He wiped inside me with some sticks like large cotton buds, and then they told me to get dressed. All through this bit I wasn't embarrassed at all. It was so impersonal – you don't feel like a real person – just someone who the doctor is examining. I suppose to him it's no more rude than looking down someone's throat.

They confirmed that I had got thrush and gave me some cream to use in the daytime and pessaries to use at night. The doctor said that my husband should use the cream as well in case he had picked it up too. I was worried about having to tell my husband because he didn't know anything about the fling I had had – and I didn't want to tell him. But the doctor explained that it's quite possible to get thrush even without having sex. What a relief!'

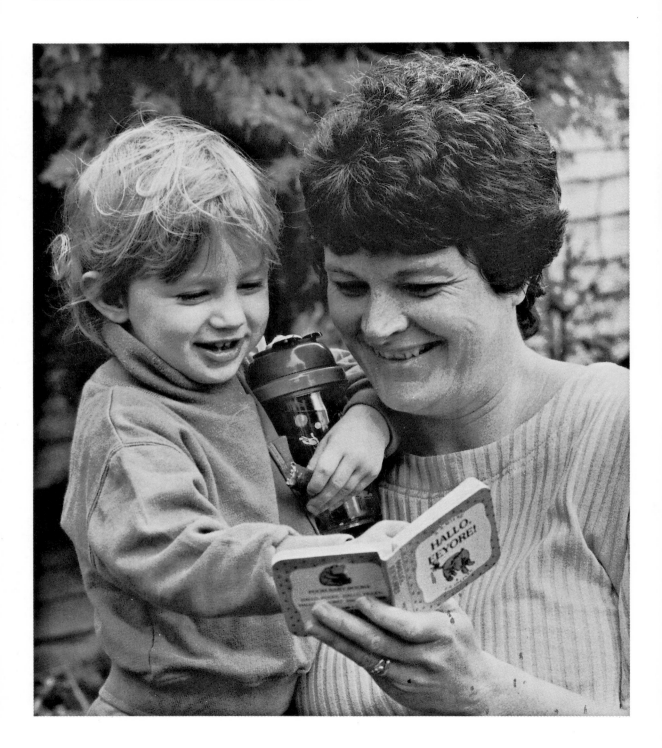

Choosing to Have Children

Society tends to assume that all women want to have children. If we say when we are young that we never want to have a family it is assumed that we will 'grow out of it'. A maternal instinct is seen as natural and normal. In fact, although most women find that they want a child, many do not. Today women have many opportunities and opting for motherhood is just one choice you can make. Women who never feel compelled to have children may be rather unusual, but their attitude is certainly not unnatural or unwomanly. Nor is it the case, as people often suspect, that they are bound to regret their decision as they grow older.

Women who decide not to have children often find themselves caught in the crossfire of other people's assumptions. People may assume that you are infertile (conversely if you are infertile people may assume you have chosen not to have children). You may feel under pressure from your friends (who may be starting families), or from your parents who want grandchildren. You may feel that people doubt that you will stick by your decision. Often employers assume that a childless woman in her thirties is a bad promotion risk because she is bound to 'get pregnant in the next few years'.

Today we have more control over whether or not we have children, and over the circumstances in which to have them, than any other generation. Effective contraception and easier access to abortion makes it easier for us to avoid unwanted pregnancies. On the other hand, attitudes to the family and access to new reproductive technologies make it possible for us to have children even if we do not live in a traditional partnership with a man.

Although some people still believe that it is only appropriate for a woman to have a child if she is married and living with her husband, alternative arrangements are becoming increasingly accepted.

The vast majority of women have their children as a consequence of, and in the context of, a heterosexual relationship with a partner with whom they share an ongoing emotional commitment. However, a growing number of women are choosing to raise their children on their own and single-parent families account for a growing proportion of families in the UK.

Are men necessary?

Some women decide from the outset that they wish to have and rear their child with as little involvement of a man as possible. Obviously, it is not possible to eradicate entirely the involvement of a man – sperm is needed after all – but a woman has various options if she is not in a steady heterosexual relationship. Some women choose to find a temporary partner specifically for the purpose of achieving a pregnancy. A few women choose to find a man, perhaps an understanding male friend, who will provide sperm with which she can inseminate herself. Other women prefer to seek artificial insemination at a licensed infertility clinic. This has the advantage that donated sperm will be from a man who has proven fertility, and has been screened to ensure that he does not carry any infections or diseases. However, many clinics are reluctant to accept single or lesbian women for treatment with donated sperm because a licensing requirement of all clinics is that they consider a resulting child's need for a father.

Is the time right?

It's hard to decide on the right time for a child. There are so many things that seem to be good reasons for deferring the moment. These include practical issues such as our careers or our financial situation, and our feelings about ourselves and our relationships. Sometimes we may feel as though we will never be ready to take on the responsibility for bringing another life into being.

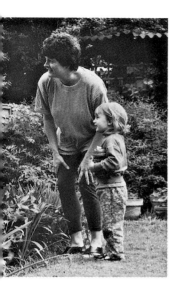

In the 1990s, women have children later. We stay single longer than past generations and have more career, education and travel opportunities. A woman is no longer seen as simply a wife and mother; it's acceptable for us to have a life outside the home at last and we take advantages of the opportunities that modern living throws our way.

Doctors still refer to any pregnant woman having her first baby over the age of 35 as an 'elderly primagravida', but it is quite common for couples to delay their family until they feel ready. Most women have their first children in their twenties, but patterns of motherhood are changing. In the last ten years the number of babies born in England and Wales to women in their early twenties dropped by almost 15,000 a year while the number born to women in their early thirties rose by almost 30,000. The number of women in their late thirties going into labour has increased by around 18,000 a year.

Advantages and disadvantages in delaying motherhood

A woman is most fertile in her early twenties and her fertility tends to decline quite rapidly after the age of 35, so, the longer you leave it, the harder you may find it to conceive. There are several reasons why fertility tends to decline with age. In the years before you reach menopause, you ovulate (release eggs) less frequently, and the eggs released may be of lower quality than those of younger women. In addition, your hormone balance may begin to change, making pregnancy less likely. Older mothers stand a higher risk of having a child with a disability as the risk of foetal abnormality increases steadily with the mother's age – and many older mothers find the early years of child rearing absolutely exhausting.

On the other hand a more mature couple may provide a more secure homelife for their children, and may be more confident and able to deal with what pregnancy and new parenthood throws at them. Techniques to detect foetal abnormalities are growing steadily more sophisticated and allow older couples to try for late pregnancy knowing that if the child has a severe detectable abnormality they can, if they choose, opt for an abortion.

Methods of antenatal diagnosis

Amniocentesis • Amniocentesis is routinely offered to pregnant women over the age of 35, and can be used to identify many chromosomal problems such as Tay-Sachs disease (which causes babies to die from progressive brain deterioration before the age of 2), Spina Bifida and Down's Syndrome. Amniocentesis involves taking fluid from the sac which surrounds the baby through a needle inserted through the abdominal wall. This fluid contains cells from the baby which are grown in a culture and then tested for chromosome abnormalities.

Amniocentesis cannot be carried out until the fifteenth or sixteenth week of pregnancy as before then the amniotic sac is too small for safe sampling. It's not quick — it usually takes at least two or three weeks to get the results.

In experienced hands amniocentesis is very safe, but there is a small risk (1 in 200) that it could trigger a miscarriage.

Chorion Villus Sampling • A small piece of the placental tissue is analysed. Because the baby and **(CVS)** placenta both develop from the same initial cells, abnormalities in the baby's cells are also likely to be present in the placenta. The cells are gathered by sucking them through a small tube which is passed through the woman's cervix or by inserting a needle through the abdominal wall. These are then tested for genetic abnormalities.

CVS can be carried out earlier than amniocentesis, usually between nine and eleven weeks, but it carries a slightly higher risk of triggering a miscarriage (around 1 in 100).

Ultrasound • Ultrasound examination can reveal certain defects of the spinal cord and abnormalities of the head and heart. Unfortunately these are difficult to spot until very late in the pregnancy – usually at about 18 or 19 weeks.

Chordocentesis (foetal blood sampling) • A needle guided by ultrasound is used to take a small sample of blood from the baby's umbilical cord. The cells are then tested as they are in CVS, but because actual foetal blood cells are obtained the results can be obtained more quickly. The risk of miscarriage is similar to that in CVS.

Foetoscopy • Certain rare liver and skin diseases can be detected by examining the baby with a special telescope-like instrument inserted into the uterus.

Maternal blood tests • Raised levels of a chemical called alphafoetolprotein (AFT) indicate that the baby is likely to have a spinal cord defect such as spina bifida. If this test is positive the woman wil! be advised to have an amniocentesis to confirm the diagnosis.

Triple test ('Barts' test) • Doctors working at London's St Bartholomew's Hospital found that women carrying babies with Down's Syndrome are more likely to have a raised level of the pregnancy hormone HCG, a lower than normal level of AFP and a raised level of a hormone called estriol.

This is an important discovery as it can identify those women under 35, who would not routinely be offered amniocentesis, who may be at risk of having a baby with Down's Syndrome. These women can then be offered an amniocentesis to confirm or overrule the diagnosis.

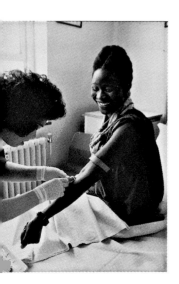

Whether or not you have tests to identify possible abnormalities is of course up to you. You may feel strongly that you want such tests either because you feel you would be able to prepare better for a child with a disability in advance of its birth, or because you feel you and your family would not be able to cope with such a baby and you would want to have an abortion.

Alternatively you may feel that you do not want such tests either because you know you would cherish your baby whatever its state of health, or because your worries about foetal handicap are fewer than your worries about the small risk of miscarriage.

If you have the tests and a foetal handicap is detected, only you can decide whether you should continue the pregnancy or opt for an abortion.

The Right Time

There is no set 'right time' to have a child. The right time for you is when you feel ready to take on all the responsibilities for bringing a new life into the world. There are some 19-year-old mothers who are more mature and capable than women in their thirties. The important thing is that a pregnancy should be 'planned and wanted'.

There are pros and cons relating to pregnancy at any age, but the vast majority of them relate to your temperament, your relationship and your lifestyle. Modern medical techniques mean that having a baby is safer than it has ever been, however old or young you are. But here are some issues to consider.

In your early twenties

pros
- you'll be at peak fertility
- you'll still be young as your child grows up
- you'll probably suffer less from tiredness in pregnancy
- you're less likely to have complications like high blood pressure
- you'll probably recover from childbirth very quickly and regain your figure faster
- the child's grandparents are likely still to be young and more able to help.

cons
- you may resent giving up your freedom to socialise
- you may not have established a career pattern
- you will have had less chance to save to see you through possible lean times ahead
- you may feel more intimidated by older doctors and midwives
- if your partner's the same age as you he may find it hard to adjust to the responsibility of being a dad.

In your late twenties

pros
- your fertility level is still high
- you are probably more confident and knowledgable about your body than when you were younger (this means you'll be more at ease when you're pregnant)
- you may be more financially secure
- you may be confident about your partner if he's been around a long time
- you may be confident about your own wants and needs
- if you have a fertility problem, there's plenty of time to sort it out.

cons
- it may be difficult to take a career break as you may have built up long-term financial commitments such as a mortgage
- you may feel that you're being pushed into motherhood because people expect it of you at this age
- you may find motherhood isolates you from your childless friends.

In your early thirties

pros
- you probably feel more confident and assertive than when you were in your twenties
- you have had more time to be sure that you want a child
- you may be more financially stable
- you probably know friends or relatives who are rearing youngsters, so you know what you're letting yourself in for.

cons
- it may be more difficult to conceive as your fertility starts to decline
- your labour might be slightly longer than it would have been in your twenties
- it will be more of a struggle to stay fit through the pregnancy
- it might take you slightly longer to recover from the birth.

In your late thirties

pros
- You will be more experienced in life and more mature
- if your partner is the same age he's also probably more mature and consequently more able to cope with the stresses of living with a pregnant woman
- you've had the chance to 'let your hair down' before the responsibility of motherhood
- you're probably more financially secure than when you were younger.

cons
- If you or your partner have a fertility problem, it may be difficult to get it sorted out before you are too old to have a child
- the risk of bearing a child with genetic defects significantly increases
- you're more likely to be at risk of high blood pressure and varicose veins
- you may feel out of place at the antenatal clinic
- you and your partner may have become set in your ways and find it more difficult to adjust to the baby
- your parents may be exhausted by their 'grandparental responsibilities'
- your friends may find it hard to adjust to your new worries about nappies, etc. when their children are well into school.

In your forties

pros
- you may find it easier to be assertive and get information out of doctors and nurses
- you may be more financially secure
- if you have children already they may by now be old enough to look after

themselves more and to help you too

- mixing with women half your age at antenatal classes will put you in touch with a younger generation.

cons
- you may find it difficult to conceive
- you may have a more difficult birth
- you are more likely to suffer from complications in pregnancy such as high blood pressure
- your labour might be slightly longer than in your early thirties
- you have significantly higher risk of bearing a child with a disability
- your child is likely to lose his or her grandparents at an early age.

Planning Your Pregnancy

It makes sense to plan your pregnancy for two reasons:

- Having a child changes your life completely
- By preparing for pregnancy you can maximise your chance of having a healthy baby.

Preconception and postconception care

Just over thirty years ago doctors did not believe that medicines taken by a pregnant woman would have an effect on her baby. They believed that the placental barrier, through which blood passes from the woman to her foetus, provided protection. Then, in the late 1950s and early 60s, the thalidomide tragedy occurred and hundreds of women all over the world bore children with severe limb deformities after taking medication to ease morning sickness.

Today we know far more about the development of the child in the womb, and we have a greater understanding of what can put it at risk and how to enhance its chances of normal development.

We know that if you are fit and well when you conceive, if you don't smoke, use recreational drugs and your intake of alcohol is moderate, your chances of having a healthy baby are improved. We also know that if a woman who has a risk of bearing a child with spina bifida increases her intake of folic acid (a B vitamin, see pages 223-226) she reduces her risk of giving birth to a child with disorders of the central nervous system, including spina bifida.

Certain foods have been shown to put pregnancies at risk because they carry bacteria which can lead to foetal death or miscarriage.

One of the problems faced by women wanting to give their pregnancies the best chance, is that it is extremely difficult to be sure when a pregnancy starts. By the time you have missed your first period the developing embryo has already passed through some of the most crucial stages of its development. This has led some doctors to suggest that every woman who is trying to conceive should consider herself pregnant in the week before her period is due and avoid exposure to anything implicated in birth defects.

This sounds like sensible advice but it places women under intense strain, especially if they do not conceive as quickly as they thought they would. Newspapers and magazines are quick to report, and sometimes sensationalise, the results of any medical research which suggests a connection, no matter how tenuous, between drugs, diet or behaviour and pregnancy outcome. As a consequence, women can often find themselves deeply anxious about their intake of vitamins, caffeine, medicines, exposure to radiation, or all kinds of hazards of daily life. It is possible that all the stress and anxiety caused by worrying about that strong cup of coffee may itself be bad for your pregnancy. You can't win. The best survival strategy is to avoid those things which have been proven to be a problem and sensibly modify your behaviour from three months before you intend to start trying for a baby.

You might want to

- Stop smoking. The birth weight of smokers' children is lower and children whose parents smoke are more prone to suffer respiratory infections and Sudden Infant Death Syndrome (Cot Death) in their first year of life.

- Cut your alcohol intake to below 14 units a week (see pages 254-255).

- Start to take supplements of folic acid to lessen your risk of bearing a child with a central nervous system disorder. The Chief Medical Officer has recommended that all women intending to become pregnant take 400mcg folic acid supplements daily. Marmite and dark green vegetables are rich in folic acid.

- Have your rubella immunity checked. This is done by a simple blood test.

- If you feel you may be at risk, you may wish to be tested for chlamydia, a sexually transmitted infection which can be symptomless in women but can cause problems in pregnancy (see page 112).

- Switch to a barrier method of contraception. Using a hormonal method of contraception right up until the time you become pregnant will not harm your baby in any way, but because it may take your body a few months to establish its natural cycle you may find it easier to date your pregnancy if you use condoms or a diaphragm for a couple of months.

- Eat sensibly. Thousands of babies are conceived by women on low-calorie or low-fat diets and they suffer no problems whatsoever. However, maintaining a good well-balanced diet (see pages 215-217) provides the best foundations for the extra energy needs of pregnancy.

Foods to avoid if you are pregnant (or trying to be)

Listeria

- Paté and certain ripened soft cheeses such as Camembert, Brie and blue veined cheeses (e.g. Gorgonzola and Stilton) may contain high levels of the bacterium listeria (listeria monocytogenes). This causes listeriosis, an illness which can result in miscarriage, stillbirth or severe illness in the newborn baby. 'Cook-chill' meals (especially ready-to-eat chicken) can also contain high levels of listeria and you should always heat them until they are piping hot, never reheat them, and never eat them cold. There is no need to worry about listeria before you know you are pregnant.

Salmonella • Raw and partly cooked eggs, poultry and raw meat can contain a bacterium called salmonella which can cause salmonellosis (often known as salmonella or salmonella gastroenteritis). This is one of the most common causes of food poisoning giving rise to sickness and diarrhoea. Although it may not have a direct effect on your unborn child it is sensible to avoid it.

Toxoplasma gondii • Raw and rare meat, unwashed vegetables and salads, and untreated goat's milk may be infected with an organism called toxoplasma gondii which causes toxoplasmosis, which in turn can cause a range of problems if passed to the unborn baby. Toxoplasmosis is also common in cat faeces.

Untreated milk (usually sold in bottles with a green top or in packets marked 'unpasteurised') may contain all manner of harmful organisms and should be avoided if you are pregnant or trying to conceive.

If you are pregnant or trying to conceive always remind your doctor of this if you need prescription medicines, and ask the advice of a pharmacist if you buy over-the-counter medicines.

Planning for the Change in Your Life

Whether you have a partner or you are single, lesbian or heterosexual, working, a student or unemployed, becoming pregnant and having a child is going to turn your life upside down.

Changes in your health

Some women seem to glide through pregnancy, remaining active until they go into labour. For others it is nine months of sheer hell. Most women experience something in between. The only thing that is certain is that you will neither be able to predict how you feel, nor what you will be capable of during pregnancy. A trouble-free first pregnancy does not guarantee

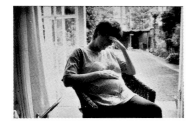

an easy second pregnancy, and conversely just because you were sick every day for the first three months of your first pregnancy does not mean you will suffer morning sickness the next time around.

Your body goes through dramatic changes during pregnancy (see below). Even in the early months, before you start to 'look pregnant', your body experiences unfamiliar surges of hormones which can make you feel unsettled and uncomfortable.

The discomforts of pregnancy

Backache (between your shoulder blades)

When to expect it
- as your breasts increase in size

How to help it
- pay attention to your posture – don't slouch.

- wear a bra that fits well. Warm baths and stretching exercises are soothing

- see a doctor if the pain is very severe when you pass water or walk – it could be a urinary tract infection.

Backache (low)

When to expect it:
- throughout pregnancy but especially in the last three months

How to help it:
- avoid high heels, use a firm mattress, pay attention to your posture. When the backache is very bad, take paracetamol

See a doctor if:
- it hurts more when you pass water or you have a history of back problems. In late pregnancy back pain which intensifies at regular intervals may be a sign of labour.

Breast tenderness

When to expect it: • in the first few months

How to help it: • wear a supportive bra

See a doctor if: • the pain is sufficiently bad to prevent you from carrying out normal activities.

Constipation

When to expect it: • after the first twelve weeks

How to help it: • eat a lot of dietary fibre (roughage) and natural laxatives (prunes, apricots)

See a doctor if: • constipation causes severe discomfort or leads to piles.

Fatigue

When to expect it: • throughout pregnancy but especially in the first and last three months

How to help it: • try to allow extra rest

See a doctor if: • it is making your life miserable.

Heartburn

When to expect it: • in the last few months

How to help it: • eat small, frequent meals, avoid anything fatty, very spicy or very cold

See a doctor if: • the pain is very severe.

Nausea

When to expect it: • from two weeks after your first missed period until week 14 or so

How to help it: • try to avoid sudden changes of position (e.g. leaping out of bed). Eat small frequent snacks of high carbohydrate foods

See a doctor if: • you are holding nothing down and think you may be at risk of dehydration.

Pubic pain

When to expect it • in the last eight weeks

How to help it: • avoid standing or walking for long periods

See a doctor if • the pain becomes unusually intense.

Shortness of breath

When to expect it: • in the last few months

How to help it: • limit your activity to whatever is comfortable

See a doctor if: • you have panic attacks where you feel you can't breathe.

Swelling

When to expect it: • A small amount of fluid retention is normal from the fifth month onwards, especially in your fingers, ankles and feet — and more noticeable at the end of the day

How to help it: • increase your fluid intake and sit with your feet raised

See a doctor if: •   swelling suddenly increases, rings feel tight, you pass water less frequently or if the swelling is accompanied by a headache. If you are unable to see a doctor straight away ring the antenatal clinic and ask to see a midwife.

Vaginal discharge

When to expect it: •   throughout pregnancy

How to help it: •   wear cotton underwear or a pantyliner.

See a doctor if: •   the discharge is a colour other than white or yellow, has an unpleasant odour or makes you feel itchy, sore or irritated.

Varicose veins

When to expect it: •   in the last three months

How to help it: •   wear support tights, take frequent rests during the day

See a doctor if: •   you get a severe pain in your legs, a red patch on the skin that is warm to touch (these can be signs of thrombosis), if your skin breaks and develops ulcers.

If you are worried

If you are worried by any symptoms at any time it is best to discuss the problem with your doctor or midwife. Never worry that they will think that you are wasting their time.

If you know what symptoms you are likely to suffer, you can plan your life around them. It does not make sense to plan major house cleaning sessions, work initiatives or active holidays when you know you are likely to feel tired and achy. You may want to avoid staying away from home early in pregnancy when you are suffering nausea. You may want to alter your work schedule so that you have more time to rest in the first and last months of pregnancy.

By recognising how you may feel you can try to take control of your life and plan around it. Clearly, it is not always possible to make the changes you would like. If you already have children they will not be less demanding because you feel tired and nauseous. However, especially early on in pregnancy when you don't yet look pregnant, it may help to explain to your family and friends how you are feeling and why you are less sparky than usual.

Changes at work

You will have to decide for yourself how much to tell your employers and colleagues about your pregnancy.

There are some advantages in announcing your pregnancy

- if you are struggling because of tiredness and morning sickness, your employers may be more sympathetic if they know that there is a reason and that it is not you being sloppy about your work

- your employers may be grateful that they have plenty of time to make arrangements for your maternity leave

- you will be able to discuss your future plans with your colleagues.

On the other hand

- you may be worried about 'counting your chickens before they hatch' especially if you are concerned that you might be at risk of miscarriage or discovering your child has a severe handicap which would cause you to have an abortion

- your employers may disapprove of your decision to have a child and interpret it as a sign that you are unserious about your career
- if your employers are particularly underhand they may try to take steps to avoid paying you maternity benefit.

Your statutory rights

From October 1994 the law will entitle all women to take maternity leave lasting for 14 weeks no matter how long they have worked for their employer. Before then your entitlement to maternity leave depended on how long you had been employed by your current employer, and how many hours you worked each week.

You have the right to time off with full pay to attend antenatal check-ups, regardless of how long you have worked. Your employer is also obliged to offer you alternative work if your usual job becomes hazardous to you or to your pregnancy. This might be the case if your job involved heavy lifting, or working with certain chemicals or drugs. In the rare case that pregnancy makes it impossible for you to continue your usual job, and there is no suitable alternative work available, your employer might be justified in dismissing you, but if this happens or if you are threatened with dismissal you should seek advice from your trade union, a Citizens' Advice Bureau or from the Equal Opportunities Commission.

You are entitled to return to work up to 29 weeks after the baby is born, providing that you have worked until the end of the twelfth week before the baby is due, that you have informed your employer at least 21 days before you leave that you are going on maternity leave, and that you intend to return to work. Your employer may request this in writing and you may have to provide a copy of your maternity certificate form.

Changes in your relationship

Approaching parenthood for the first time in your life can certainly be pretty terrifying. Suddenly you find that you are faced with the daunting responsibility for another completely dependent and very demanding human being.

There are no longer just two of you, and this in itself can be difficult to get used to. You may find that in the months following the birth of your child you find it hard to cope with conflicting demands, responsibilities and your own feelings for each other. Your partner may feel pushed to one side if he feels he takes second place to the new baby. You may find it difficult to respond as a lover and friend when your days are so dominated by motherhood. The first months of family life are a challenging time for everyone.

There is no magic elixir to soothe away the problems. If you can, you may find it helps to try to set aside a small amount of time each day, even if it is just 15 minutes, when you talk together. You may find that your relationships with friends and colleagues change too. Through antenatal classes you will acquire a new circle of acquaintances and perhaps new friends with whom you will have a lot in common. Your existing friends, especially those who do not have children may worry that you will drift away from them as you become absorbed in motherhood. Try to understand any tensions that may arise because of these fears and make an effort to keep in touch with those who have loved and supported you before the pregnancy.

Changes to your finances

Having a child knocks a serious dent in your finances. Time off work, if you have a job, coincides with increased expenditure to prepare for the new addition to your life.

State benefits are rather low, but they can alleviate some hardship and it makes sense to take advantage of them.

In the UK *all* pregnant women have the right to free dental treatment on the NHS while pregnant and for a year after birth. You also receive free NHS prescriptions while you are pregnant and for you and your child immediately after a birth.

Pregnant women on income support can also claim

- free milk tokens
- free vitamin tablets while you are pregnant and breast feeding, vitamin drops for your child until he or she reaches the age of 5
- vouchers for spectacles
- fares to and from hospital
- a lump sum maternity payment.

All mothers can claim Child Benefit, and if you are in low-paid, full-time work you may be able to claim Family Credit.

Getting Pregnant

Human conception is a chancy business. A farmer expects his animals to have at least one offspring as a result of a mating. Humans are not quite so predictable. Despite being, as a species, fertile enough to be the most populous animal on the planet, our individual fertility is quite low. A fertile couple making love at the most fertile time of the woman's cycle only has one chance in four of conceiving. This is despite the fact that when an averagely fertile man ejaculates he deposits 60 to 100 million sperm in his partner's vagina – enough to impregnate every woman in the UK. Some studies suggest that if a fertile couple make love daily, it will take them on average three months for the woman to become pregnant, while if they make love ten times or fewer during the month it may take at least six months.

Egg being released
Fallopian tube

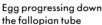

Ovary

Vagina

Egg progressing down
the fallopian tube

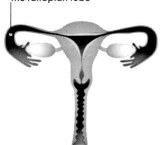

Egg

Sperm being
ejaculated

Penis

Egg being fertilised

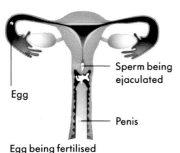

Sperm

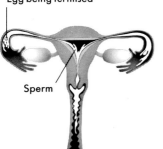

When you are most fertile

The most fertile days of the month are those *directly before you ovulate* as it gives the sperm the chance to get into peak position in the fallopian tubes before the egg is released.

If you have regular periods you can expect to ovulate between 12 and 16 days before the due date of your next period. If you are sensitive to the effects of your monthly cycle, you may be able to tell that you are about to ovulate from the following signs:

- the texture of your vaginal secretions change to feel slippery and wet like raw egg white.
- some women feel an ache or pain in their groin (known as *mittelschmerz*) as an egg is released.

You can also detect when and if you are ovulating by using a home ovulation test. This works by detecting a sudden surge in the level of luteinizing hormone which triggers ovulation (LH). Once you've detected this surge you know that the next two to three days are your most fertile.

For fertilisation to occur, the egg, once released from the ovary, has to be wafted in the fallopian tube along which it must pass into the womb. It is here that it meets a lurking sperm to fertilise it. Recent research shows that as many as four eggs out of every ten released fail to make it into the fallopian tube. And out of the 60 per cent that make it 15 per cent of the eggs are defective in some way and can't be fertilised.

There is no hard evidence to suggest that any particular sexual positions make conception easier than others. Pillows under the woman's buttocks may feel nice, but they are not a fertility aid; neither is the advice sometimes given to lie in bed for 30 minutes after intercourse. It's normal for semen to leak out of the vagina and this doesn't affect a woman's

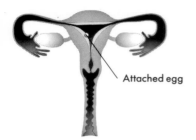

Attached egg

chances of conceiving. On the contrary, it should be taken as an assurance that your partner has a normal volume of seminal fluid.

If the egg is fertilised it continues its journey down to the womb where it burrows into the specially prepared womb lining. If it isn't fertilised, the egg is absorbed into the woman's body and the womb lining breaks down and bleeds away as a period.

A missed period

For most women, a missed period is the first sign of pregnancy. However, this isn't always the case. If the embryo implants in the womb lining, extra blood vessels develop around it which can cause bleeding in around 20 per cent of women. Many women mistake this bleeding for a period and so when they eventually realise that they are pregnant, they think the gestation is a month younger than it really is.

Pregnancy symptoms

Even before a woman has a strong suspicion that she is pregnant, she may experience the following symptoms:

- Tiredness, especially early in the morning and late in the evening. This is owing to the pregnancy consuming the body's energy resources.
- Breast tenderness occurs very frequently and is also a response to hormone surges.
- Nausea commonly starts slightly later, from about sixteen days after ovulation, as the body responds to a surge in the pregnancy hormones.
- Mood swings and tearfulness for unexplained reasons is common.

None of these symptoms is conclusive, in fact many are experienced by women prior to their period. But if you experience any of them – and a delayed period – you should be on 'pregnancy alert'.

Many pregnancy tests, available 'over the counter' at your local pharmacy, can give you a result shortly after your period is due. They work by detecting the pregnancy hormone, *human chorionic gonadotrophin* (HCG), which is detectable in the urine within seven days of fertilisation. All the tests on sale are accurate, but they are not cheap and you may prefer to have a free test carried out at your doctor's surgery or family planning clinic. However, these tests are often a cheaper, less sensitive kind and you may have to wait until your period is two weeks late before having the test.

When Things Go Wrong

Subfertility

If you have difficulty conceiving

Out of every ten couples having unprotected sex at the right time of the month, eight will become pregnant within a year, a further couple will conceive within two years and one couple will probably need medical help. Most doctors won't even consider referring you for infertility investigations unless you have been trying to conceive for two years if you are under 35, and one year if you are older. If you have been trying to conceive for more than a year most doctors will regard you as 'subfertile'.

The time between realising that there may be a problem and waiting for investigations to start is extremely frustrating. Many experts believe that apart from making love at the 'right time of the month' there is little you can do. However, some factors have been linked to subfertility and it makes sense to avoid them:

- cut down on alcohol and smoking. Both have been linked to fertility problems in men and women
- stick to a balanced diet. Now is not the time to count calories unless you

are clinically overweight (in which case it's advisable to try to get as near to your normal weight as possible)

- encourage your partner to wear boxer shorts and looser trousers rather than Y-fronts and tight jeans, as sperm production is best when testicles are cool.

Try to remember that sex is for fun as well as fertility. Many couples, anxious to conceive, end up with all manner of sexual and emotional problems because they feel they have 'to perform to order'. Nothing is more of a turn-off than feeling you *have* to make love because it's 'that time of the month'.

Doubts about fertility can make both halves of a partnership feel insecure. A woman who has always assumed she will one day be a mother, can feel as though her whole role in life is under threat. A man who has always assumed he would be able to father children often feels inadequate and 'less of a man'. Just at the time when you both need reassurance from each other may be the time when you are most confused about your own feelings.

Infertility

Infertility is one of the biggest cons nature can pull. You spend years carefully using contraception to protect against accidental pregnancies, only to find out that you needn't have bothered after all.

A successful conception relies on a healthy egg being released and penetrated by a healthy sperm within twenty-four hours. It then has to travel down the fallopian tubes to implant in the womb. At any stage things can snarl up. Experts estimate that 40 per cent of healthy eggs fail to make it into the fallopian tubes and a quarter of those that do and are successfully penetrated by a sperm fail to implant in the womb. Looked at in that way it seems extraordinary that anyone ever gets pregnant!

A decade ago, doctors estimated that one couple in ten was infertile. Now they believe as many as one in six will need help to conceive within a reasonable time.

Common causes of infertility (women)

Failure to ovulate

Often caused by
- polycystic ovary syndrome
- physical damage to the ovaries perhaps as a result of scarring after the removal of ovarian cysts, or radiation therapy after cancer
- sometimes, for reasons not yet understood, the woman produces a perfectly good egg but the ovary fails to release it
- severe stress, perhaps as a consequence of bereavement or redundancy, has also been associated with a temporary failure to ovulate.

Damaged fallopian tubes

Often caused by
- tubal scarring, a common consequence of infections like gonorrhoea or more commonly chlamydia
- inflammation of the abdominal cavity or bowels can spread to the tubes
- previous ectopic pregnancies
- endometriosis
- congenital defects.

Abnormal uterus

Often caused by
- fibroids or polyps (non-cancerous growths in the womb)
- congenital abnormalities
- adhesions (where the internal walls stick together)

Problem cervical mucus

- Hormonal factors may mean that insufficient 'fertile' mucus is produced to create favourable conditions for the sperm just before ovulation.

Common causes of infertility (men)

Problem testicles

Often caused by
- a previous hard blow (perhaps a sporting injury)
- a previous severe mumps infection
- previous damage to the blood supply (perhaps due to serious twisting)
- failure of the testicles to descend into the scrotum when young
- congenital defect (likely to be chromosomal)
- blockages in the tubes
- retrograde ejaculation

Abnormal sperm

Low sperm count and poor motility are often caused by
- hormonal problems
- varicocele (enlarged veins which overheat the testes)
- a current or previous infection

Immunological problems

- For unknown reasons, men form antibodies which attack their own sperm

Sexual difficulties

Such as
- impotence
- premature ejaculation

Anatomical abnormalities

These are extremely rare but include
- a condition when the tube that carries the sperm to the end of the erect penis stops short

- absence of the vas deferens or otherwise poorly developed testicles.

Environmental factors

All the following can affect sperm quality and quantity

- smoking
- possibly alcohol
- obesity
- drugs — including prescription drugs such as some antidepressants, those used to treat high blood presure and antimalarial products.

The tests

Initial tests can be carried out by a GP

For the woman

- A blood test can detect if you ovulate

For the man

- A sperm analysis can measure the quality and quantity of sperm. There may be a problem if:

- the volume of semen is less than 2ml or greater than 5ml

- there are fewer than 20 million sperm per ejaculation

- fewer than 40 per cent of sperm are moving and fewer than 65 per cent look normal under a microscope

Secondary tests carried out at an infertility clinic

For both

- post-coital test. Sample of fluid is taken from the woman's cervix six to eighteen hours after sex. This can show how the sperm behaves in the woman's cervical mucus. It might reveal if the woman is producing antibodies which attack the sperm

For the woman

- a Hysterosalpingogram (HSG) is an X-ray of the uterus and fallopian tubes following the injection of a little dye through the opening of the cervix. This reveals valuable information about the condition of the uterus and fallopian tubes. It's painless

- a laparoscopy is usually carried out under general anaesthetic. A thin telescope is inserted into the abdominal cavity through a small incision in the navel. Through this the surgeon can inspect the uterus, the ovaries and the outside of the fallopian tubes

- if there's a suspect ovulatory problem the clinic will carry out more detailed hormonal tests

- a chromosome test can detect if there is a problem which would lead to the production of abnormal eggs.

For the man

- hormone tests may reveal a problem that leads to a low sperm count

- antibody tests might reveal if he produces antibodies which destroy his own sperm

a chromosome test might show if there is a genetic reason for problem sperm.

Treatments

Low-tech 'do it yourself' fertility aids

For both partners there are general health measures you can take to boost fertility

- lose excess weight
- stop smoking and drinking alcohol

For the man • keep testicular temperature as low as possible by avoiding tight trousers or underpants. Some specialists advocate dangling the testicles in cold water for ten minutes a day

• Vitamin C and E supplements are sometimes recommended.

For the woman • ensure that you make love frequently, during, and just before your fertile period.

Assisted Conception Techniques

For the woman • tubal surgery to repair damaged fallopian tubes. Success rates depend on the surgeon's skill but the operation is usually only successful in about 10 per cent of cases.

For both • artificial insemination with partner's or donor sperm. A simple procedure where sperm is placed in the vagina to coincide with ovulation

• intrauterine insemination bypasses the cervix and places the sperm directly into the uterine cavity. Works for about a third of couples if repeated over several months

• in vitro fertilisation (IVF) involves egg and sperm collection followed by fertilisation in a laboratory before the embryo is replanted in the uterus. Success rates vary, with the more experienced clinics claiming 25-30 per cent success

• gamete intra-fallopian transfer (GIFT) involves eggs and sperm being collected from both partners. They are mixed together and returned to the fallopian tubes before fertilisation. Recent studies suggest it's about half as efficient as IVF.

Other techniques • Other techniques, known as micromanipulation techniques, involve altering the egg itself so as to make it easier for a sperm to fertilise it

- subzonal insemination (SUZI). The injection of sperm into the egg itself

- partial zonal dissection (PZD). The rupturing of the egg cell wall to allow the sperm easier access.

Such techniques are still at the stage where they are better described as 'medical experiments' rather than practical treatment options. Only about 5 per cent of couples undergoing SUZI will achieve a successful pregnancy and the technique is only available at a tiny number of clinics.

Richard, a 40-year-old architect and 32-year-old Penny, a secretary, were referred to a specialist after three years of trying for a baby. At first it was assumed that the problem lay with Penny. Richard was only asked to produce a sperm sample after Penny had been subjected to blood tests to check her hormone levels, ovulation tests to check that she was releasing eggs and several vaginal examinations. When Richard's semen was analysed doctors found that he was producing only a small quantity of poor-quality sperm. They concluded that IVF might help, but a cycle failed to result in any fertilised eggs and they were told there was probably nothing to be gained from trying again.

Richard's story

'I was devastated by the test results. I would never have believed I could feel so inadequate. Suddenly you start looking at every man you meet in a new way. I hold an executive position in a top company, and I always thought I was in control of my life. The guy on reception, for example, is on a salary a fraction of mine but he's managed to have three children.

It's awful knowing that I can't give Penny what I know she most wants. I was brought up to believe that men provide for women, and so I feel I'm not only letting her down, I'm letting myself down too. Every time I see her cry, or I sense that she's depressed, I feel responsible. There doesn't seem to be anyone to talk to. I haven't been able to bring myself to admit to my friends that I've a problem. I suppose it's because there's still so much stigma attached to the subject. Since I was told I couldn't father a child it seems to have become the most important thing in the world.

I wasn't sure about joining the IVF programme. I knew the success rate was low. But the worst side of it was seeing Penny suffer so much. I felt I was having an easy ride although I was responsible for the problem. Penny had to inhale hormones every four hours for nearly a month to shut down her natural cycle of egg production. Then she had to have injections every day for ten days to stimulate eggs to grow. She also had to undergo an operation to have eggs removed so that they could be mixed with my sperm. If the eggs had fertilised (which they didn't) there would have been another operation to put them into her womb. All I had to do was masturbate into a jar. It was one of the most degrading experiences of my life, but compared to what Penny went through, it was nothing.

I can't describe how I felt when the doctor told us that there was no chance of Penny having a child using my sperm, but she stood a good chance of conceiving using donor sperm. I don't know if I could cope with that.'

Penny's story

'It took a few days for the test results to sink in and then the numbness turned to grief and I felt as though someone had died. That was the worst time. I wanted to talk about how I felt, but I couldn't talk to Richard because I could see on his face how painful it was for him. I felt entirely alone. Usually I cry on my mother's shoulder if I can't turn to Richard, but how can your mother understand what it feels like to be infertile?

I'm aware that Richard is acutely embarrassed about the problem and he *really doesn't want our friends to know. I suppose this in itself has been a strain. I don't want to betray him, but it means we have to pretend that we're childless through choice. In my heart I've never given up hoping that one day something will happen.*

In many ways it seems more difficult knowing that I can have a child in the abstract but I can't have Richard's child. I feel I've had to choose between motherhood and the man I love. The specialist seemed quite surprised when I was adamant that I wouldn't consider donor sperm, that I wanted our child. Sometimes I worry about how I'll feel when I get towards the end of my fertile years. I'm worried that I may grow to resent Richard, but I think we can handle it. In some ways I think the experience has bonded us more strongly together. When he counselled us after the IVF failed, our doctor warned that infertility problems often break marriages, and I can understand how that can happen.'

Ectopic Pregnancy

Sometimes, instead of travelling down the fallopian tube and implanting in the uterus, as it should, a fertilised egg implants somewhere else – usually in one of the fallopian tubes, but occasionally elsewhere in the abdominal cavity. Sometimes this happens because the fallopian tube is already damaged or scarred as a result of an infection or condition like endometriosis.

Ectopic pregnancies are always problematic because if the embryo continues to grow it will rupture the tube which may result in a haemorrhage. Occasionally the embryo may stop developing and be absorbed back into the body.

Sometimes it is difficult for doctors to diagnose an ectopic pregnancy and it is sometimes mistaken for appendicitis, or the threatened miscarriage of a normal pregnancy. You may or may not feel pain in the area where the embryo is growing. Some women, but not all, have a positive pregnancy test and some of the symptoms of early pregnancy such as tiredness, enlarged tender breasts and nausea. Usually there will be at least one missed menstrual period, followed by slight bleeding and pain, but even this is not always the case. Some women continue to have periods, experience no other symptoms and their problem is not diagnosed until the tube ruptures. This usually occurs between the eighth and twelfth weeks of pregnancy depending on whether the embryo has implanted in the narrower or broader end of the fallopian tube. A ruptured tube occurs in about a third of all ectopic pregnancies. Sometimes it causes sudden acute pain and bleeding sufficient enough to cause the woman to collapse; more often the rupture is a gradual process with intermittent bleeding and pain.

Danger signs

- a sudden sharp or persistent pain in the lower abdomen
- a pain that feels as though it is under one of your shoulder blades
- irregular bleeding or staining and abdominal pain following a very light or late period.

If you are sexually active and you experience any of the above you should seek medical treatment immediately, and explain that you think you may be suffering from an ectopic pregnancy.

Treatment depends on where the embryo has implanted and whether there is any infection.

If your doctor suspects you have an ectopic pregnancy you will be admitted to hospital for an examination of your pelvic cavity and fallopian tubes. This will be carried out using a fine telescope. If an ectopic pregnancy is confirmed the surgeon will carry out a laparotomy, an incision into the lower abdomen to remove the embryo. Often a section of the fallopian tube will need to be removed and sometimes the ovary too.

Unfortunately an ectopic pregnancy will usually have a negative effect on your future fertility as it usually causes permanent damage to one of your fallopian tubes. However, your other tube will not have been affected and will still work normally, so if you do not wish to conceive you will need to continue to use contraception. Sadly, women who have suffered one ectopic pregnancy have a higher risk of another than women who have never suffered this problem.

Miscarriage

The loss of a wanted pregnancy is one of the most painful experiences a woman can suffer no matter what stage of pregnancy the miscarriage occurs. An early miscarriage is not necessarily less traumatic than a later miscarriage. Doctors, especially hospital doctors, still tend to use the term 'abortion' to describe the condition although for most of us abortion is understood to be a deliberate termination of a pregnancy, whereas miscarriage is an involuntary termination.

Medical terms used to refer to miscarriage

Spontaneous abortion • This is the general medical term for what we normally know as abortion and it is used to refer to the expulsion of the embryo or foetus from the uterus before the twenty-fourth week of pregnancy. The embryo is referred to as a foetus from the eighth week of pregnancy.

Stillbirth • From the twenty-fourth week, if the baby is born and shows no signs of life it is referred to as a stillbirth.

Threatened abortion • This indicates that the pregnancy might be in danger. The woman may be experiencing some period-like cramps and bleeding, spotting or staining from the vagina. At this stage it will be impossible for a doctor to tell whether or not these are the first signs of a miscarriage. Many women who have bleeding in early pregnancy go on to have normal pregnancies. Doctors regard cramping as more worrying than bleeding.

Inevitable abortion   •   This is used to describe a situation where the cervix has opened. When this happens nothing can be done to save the pregnancy. The woman usually experiences an increase in pain and bleeding.

Incomplete abortion   •   Sometimes not all of the 'products of conception' are lost during a miscarriage and sections of the uterine lining or the placenta may remain in the uterus. If this happens usually the bleeding will continue until it is removed surgically and there is a risk of infection if this is not done.

Missed abortion   •   Sometimes the embryo or foetus is not expelled from the woman's body even though it has died. This can be extremely confusing for the woman, especially in early pregnancy, because her symptoms such as morning sickness may stop but there may be no bleeding. Sometimes a spontaneous miscarriage may happen at a later date, but the contents of the womb may have to be removed surgically.

Recurrent abortion   •   A woman is understood to be suffering from this problem when she has three or more miscarriages.

Septic abortion   •   This is used to describe an infection of the uterus following a miscarriage or abortion.

Early miscarriage

Miscarriage is still largely a medical mystery. Most are unexplained and the vast majority of women who suffer one, even two miscarriages then go on to carry a normal pregnancy to term. Because of this doctors will not normally even try to investigate to find a reason for an early miscarriage until a woman has had at least three.

Early miscarriages may occur either as a consequence of a problem with the developing embryo or foetus, or a problem with the mother. Statistics suggest that possibly as many as 60 per cent of early miscarriages take place because the embryo has a chromosomal abnormality. The real percentage may be even higher as some abnormalities are not yet detectable. These are just 'one-off' problems with a particular sperm or egg rather than one which is likely to be repeated. Sometimes, even though there is no chromosomal problem, the anatomical structure of the embryo may fail to develop normally and this may lead to miscarriage.

Some infections and illnesses (such as listeriosis, rubella, and some sexually transmitted infections such as chlamydia) can trigger early miscarriage but sometimes the problem can be the way a woman's body responds to the pregnancy. Progesterone and HCG are important to the development and sustenance of a pregnancy and a woman may be unable to sustain her pregnancy if she does not produce sufficient quantities. Some doctors advocate hormonal supplements if a woman has repeated miscarriages, but studies are inconclusive as to whether this treatment makes a difference.

When a woman has recurrent early miscarriages she and her partner may be investigated to see if there is an immunological cause. In a normal pregnancy, the woman's body recognises the embryo as a foreign body and triggers a complicated response to prevent it from being rejected. It seems that in some women, especially if she and her partner have very similar tissue types or chromosomal structures, the woman's body may not recognise the embryo as a foreign body until it is too late for it to be protected. In cases where this is a problem treatment is sometimes available to stimulate the appropriate response.

The symptoms of an early miscarriage

- Bleeding – which can vary between a brownish discharge, spotting or a period-like loss. The bleeding may keep stopping and starting or it may be heavy. It is important to remember that bleeding in early pregnancy does not necessarily mean that a miscarriage will follow, and some studies suggest that as many as one woman in five has a certain amount of bleeding in early pregnancy.

- Pains or backache, often similar to period pains, sometimes more severe, are experienced by many women. Again these symptoms are also common in normal healthy pregnancies.

- Reductions in the signs of pregnancy may indicate a problem. Some women find that their breasts no longer feel so tender or their morning sickness lessens. This is particularly confusing especially if it is your first pregnancy and you do not know how you should expect to feel.

- There is virtually nothing you or your doctor can do to prevent a miscarriage. Some doctors recommend bed rest but there is no evidence that it makes a difference to the outcome. A pregnancy test to measure the levels of pregnancy hormone is an unreliable indication of whether the pregnancy is still viable because it can take days for the levels to drop even after the miscarriage has taken place or the embryo or foetus has died. An ultrasound scan may be able to indicate whether there is evidence of a foetal or embryonic heartbeat or whether the embryo is situated normally in the uterus, but even these are not foolproof as the foetal sac may be obscured.

- If the miscarriage is inevitable, most doctors will try to avoid surgical intervention if at all possible and will prefer to wait for a few days to see if your body clears itself before arranging an operation to empty the uterus. If the miscarriage has not occurred but a scan shows without doubt that there is an empty sac or that the fetus is dead then most doctors would probably advocate an operation. When medical intervention is necessary it takes the same form as in a voluntary abortion (see pages 78-83).

Later miscarriage

Miscarriages which occur after 16 weeks are much less common than early miscarriages. They can occur for a variety of reasons and do not necessarily mean that future pregnancies will be jeopardised.

Later miscarriages are sometimes caused by anatomical abnormalities in the mother, for example the structure of the uterus or the presence of polyps (see pages 53-54) may prevent the foetus from developing properly or the entrance to the uterus may not be sufficiently strong to support the developing fetus (cervical incompetence). These problems can usually be rectified by surgical intervention so that future pregnancies are unaffected.

Some antenatal tests slightly increase the risk of miscarriage and if you are pregnant and considering such tests you should ensure your doctor discusses the risks with you (see pages 127-130).

Late miscarriages are particularly distressing as they involve the woman in an experience very much like labour. Women who miscarry from 19 weeks (and sometimes earlier) are likely to produce milk which not only means that breasts become extremely painful but also reinforces the sense of loss. Some doctors will provide medication to prevent this.

The emotional impact of a miscarriage at any stage of pregnancy can be devastating for both partners. It is a true bereavement.

Surviving Motherhood

Motherhood affects your health and well-being until your children leave home and in many cases far beyond even then.

When you have a child you bring into your life a new source of pleasure, delight and stimulation, and also a new source of stresses, strains, annoyance and anxiety. The specific forms that the tensions take change as the children grow, but they never really go away. Each stage of your son's or daughter's development, from infant to adolescent, has its own trials and joys.

A mother's wisdom

'I woke up five months into my second pregnancy and thought I can't go through with it again. It wasn't the thought of labour that terrified me it was the memory of my first child taking an entire year before she slept through a complete night.'

'I thought I would break my heart when he first started school – he seemed so small and vulnerable. Then I realised that it was me that was feeling small and vulnerable. Tom came dashing through the gates proud of his new model and hand in hand with a new friend. I felt as though I wasn't needed any more. I remember sitting in the kitchen on the second day thinking what on earth am I going to do with myself?'

'The teenage years are definitely the worst. It seems as though there aren't any rules any more. I'm scared of being too hard on her, and even more scared of being too soft. Everyone wants to give you advice, but it's all different.'

'I'm sure it's easier to bring up boys than girls. They can't get pregnant for one thing.'

'I'm sure girls are easier to handle than boys. They don't feel under so much pressure to run with the crowd and prove themselves.'

'Every mother I know has a multiple personality. Sometimes I think motherhood must be a kind of mental illness like a multiple personality disorder. You end up balancing so many different demands it's hard to remember who the real you is.'

'Sometimes I'm desperate for someone to want me for being just me – Joan – not for being a mother, wife or worker.'

'Motherhood is definitely a kind of madness – but the kids grow out of it and so do you!'

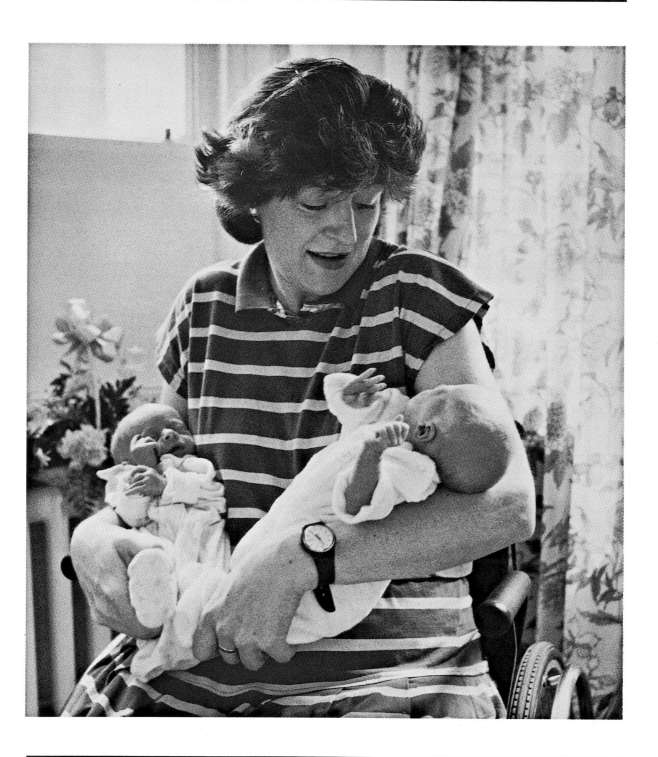

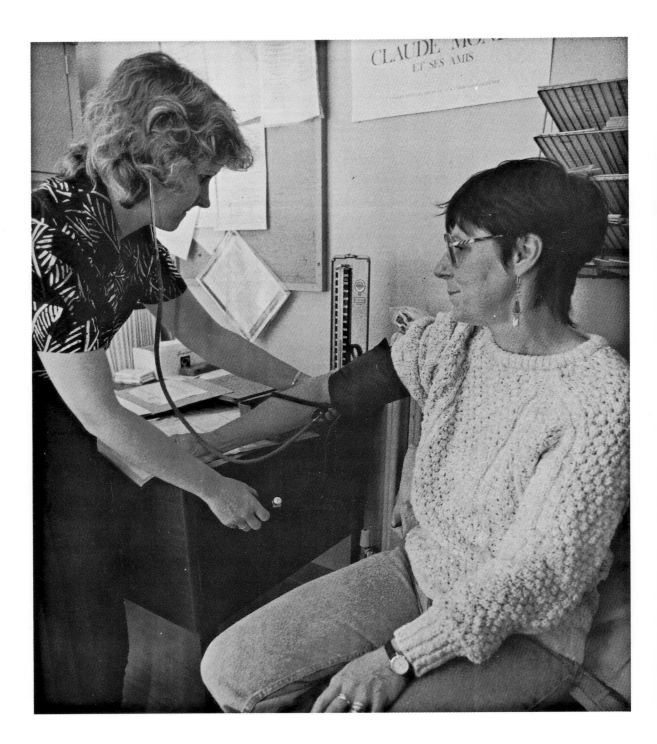

Cancer

What is cancer?

This section considers some of the most common cancers in women. They are particularly important because there are steps you can take to prevent them; or there are tests to help you detect them early, thus greatly increasing your chance of recovery. After heart disease, breast cancer and lung cancer are the leading causes of death for women under 65. Skin cancer and cervical cancer also affect a large number of women, many of them young.

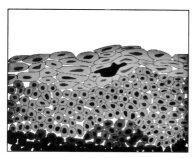

Cancer can start from a single abnormal cell

Cancer is not a single disease but a type of disease. There are over 200 different cancers, each occurring in its own way. What they have in common is that they all start with a change in the normal make-up of a cell. The division of normal cells is carefully controlled. But abnormal cells divide in an uncontrolled manner, and seem not to know when to stop. How quickly a cancer grows and spreads can be very different for each individual cancer.

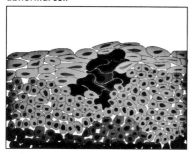

The abnormal cell divides to produce a tumour

A cluster of abnormal cells is called a *tumour* or *primary growth*. Not all tumours are cancers, however. There are two types of tumour – benign and malignant.

Benign tumours are not cancers. They usually don't need treatment. But, if they do, they can be removed by simple surgery.

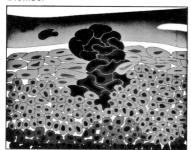

Cancer cells break away from the tumour and travel through the bloodstream to other parts of the body

Malignant tumours are cancers and can be dangerous. They can invade nearby parts of the body and may stop cells there from working properly. Cells from malignant tumours can break away and travel – through the bloodstream, for instance – to other parts of the body. There they settle, forming new colonies of abnormal cells. These are called secondary growths.

The whole process is known as metastasis. It is one of the main features of cancer, and is what makes it dangerous. It's important to spot cancers early, before metastasis has happened. With many types of cancer, early detection can widen your treatment options and greatly improve the chances of successful treatment. The first step is to develop personal awareness of changes in your body, so that any worrying symptoms can be taken to your doctor early.

The most important symptoms to look out for

- a lump anywhere in your body, e.g. in your breast
- a change in a skin mole
- a sore that does not heal
- a persistent cough or hoarseness
- persistent indigestion or difficulty swallowing
- vomiting or coughing up blood
- change in normal bowel habit, such as persistent diarrhoea or constipation
- any bleeding in the urine or bowel movement and any abnormal vaginal bleeding
- unexplained weight loss
- unexplained loss of appetite

Lung cancer

The incidence of lung cancer among women in the UK has increased greatly over the past few decades, particularly for older women, and in some areas has overtaken breast cancer as the most common cancer. Smoking causes about seven out of ten cases of lung cancer in women, and the rise in incidence has been thanks to dramatic changes in smoking behaviour among women in the last fifty years (see Smoking, pages 236-251).

Breast cancer

What is it?

- The breast is made up of fatty tissue, milk ducts and milk-producing sacs.

The lymph system drains the breast into lymph nodes in the armpit and under the breast bone. Cancer cells may start to grow in the milk ducts or sacs and then spread into the lymphatic system. While the tumour is only within the breast, it is fairly easily removed. Once it spreads to the armpit and more widely round the body, it becomes more difficult to treat, so early detection is vital.

Who is at risk ? • One woman in twelve in the UK develops breast cancer. It is by far the most common type of cancer in women, and England and Wales together have one of the highest rates in the world. Breast cancer is the second commonest cause of death among women under the age of 65, after circulatory diseases, although death rates seem to be falling. The likelihood of developing breast cancer increases with age, and it is very rare in women under 30. One-third of women are in their seventies when they develop breast cancer. African-Caribbean and Asian women have a lower incidence. Breast feeding seems to protect against developing breast cancer.

A number of factors affects your chance of getting breast cancer, although just because these apply to you does not mean you will get it

• never having children, or having your first child after the age of 30 increases your risk.

• starting your periods early (before 12) or finishing them late (after 50) gives you a slightly higher risk.

• if your mother or sister has had breast cancer, then your risk is doubled.

• being overweight increases your risk.

• a high-fat diet may be linked to breast cancer. In countries such as Japan, with low fat intakes, the incidence is low, but rises dramatically for Japanese women who move elsewhere and have a Western diet.

• using HRT for ten years or more seems to increase your risk of breast cancer, although some experts do not agree.

• using the oral contraceptive pill before the age of 25, and continuing to use it for more than four years may increase your risk, although the evidence is not clear.

• the older you are, the greater your chance of developing breast cancer.

NHS breast screening

What is it ? • Breast screening, or mammography, is an X-ray examination of the breasts. It can help to find small changes in the breast before there are any other signs or symptoms of cancer. If these changes are found at an early stage, there is a good chance of a successful recovery. Today, with early detection and effective treatment, around 80 per cent of women with breast cancer will recover.

Who is it for ? • Free breast screening is being offered by the NHS to all women between the ages of 50 and 64. In order to be invited for screening, you need to be registered with a GP and it is important that your doctor has your up-to-date address at all times. If you are under the age of 50, you will not receive an invitation for breast screening. Breast cancer is not so common in women of this age group, and the general screening of women under 50 has not yet proved to be helpful in reducing the number of deaths from cancer. However, if you are worried about any breast problem, you should go to your doctor who will refer you for a specialist opinion if necessary.

If you are 65 or over you will not automatically be invited for screening, but you will be screened if you request it. You should talk to your doctor if you want to find out more about this, or contact your local screening centre.

The Breast Screening Service has been running throughout the UK since 1990, and every woman between the ages of 50 and 64 should have been screened in the first three years of operation. If you are in this age group and have not received an invitation for screening, ask your doctor about the service.

What happens ? • The screening centre will be in a hospital or clinic, or it may be a mobile unit. When you arrive, a nurse or radiographer will explain things to you and ask a few questions, and you should feel free to ask about anything you are unsure of.

You will undress down to the waist, and first one and then the other breast will be compressed between two special plates and an X-ray taken of each. It may feel a bit uncomfortable, but it only lasts a few minutes. Try to relax by breathing deeply.

After you have had the mammogram, you will be told how and roughly when you will hear the results – it's important to be clear about this before you leave.

Getting the results • Most women will receive a normal result, and will then be recalled automatically in three years' time for another test.

Don't be too alarmed if you are called back for a repeat test straightaway. Sometimes a test needs to be repeated before you can get the results because of a technical problem with the test, for example with the film. Or the appearance of the X-ray may suggest the need for further investigation, which turns out to be nothing significant. If this is the case, you will be told there is nothing to worry about, and recalled in three years' time.

What if they find • If the result of your mammogram is positive, you will be called back to
cancer? discuss further specialist treatment needed. This will obviously be a very traumatic time, and you need to find support from friends and family who are able to share your situation. A number of different treatment options may be offered, including surgery, radiotherapy and chemotherapy, or a combination of them.

Radiotherapy • This is treatment with high-energy X-rays to the breast and surrounding lymph nodes. A full course of radiotherapy may be anything from one to twenty treatments.

Chemotherapy • This involves the use of drugs to control cancer cells, some of which may have spread elsewhere in the body.

Surgery • Surgery may involve a lumpectomy, which is the removal of the lump and a small area of breast tissue surrounding it. Or you may need a mastectomy to remove part or all of your breast, sometimes with lymph nodes and part or all of the tissue from the armpit.

Getting help • It may help to talk to someone who has been through a similar experience and has come through it. Breast Cancer Care is a national organisation offering free help, information and support and free publications to women with breast cancer or other breast-related problems. It operates a volunteer network nationwide, where helpers with personal experience of breast surgery will telephone or visit you if you need information or support. There is also a prosthesis service, which can give you information about getting a prosthesis on the NHS, through retail outlets or through Breast Cancer Care.

Be breast aware

It is important that you know the normal look and feel of your breasts. It is not necessary to perform a ritual breast examination at a certain time in your monthly cycle each month. What is more helpful is to be aware of your breasts at all times, to look out for any unusual signs, and report them to your doctor straightaway. Of particular concern is any unusual change in the outline, shape or size of the breast, puckering or dimpling of the skin, a lump or thickening in the breast or armpit, any flaking of the skin, discharge from the nipple or any unusual pain or discomfort. A change in position of the nipple – if it is pulled in or pointing upwards – should also be checked. Use a mirror, and watch for any changes when you raise your arms.

Before you reach the menopause, you may notice that your breasts feel different at different times in your cycle. In the days leading up to a period, the milk-producing tissue becomes active, and your breasts may feel tender or lumpy, especially near the armpits.

After the menopause, your breasts may feel soft, less firm and not lumpy. If you have had a hysterectomy, you may notice the same changes in your breasts during each month until you reach the time when your periods would have ceased.

If you do notice any changes, you should go to your doctor without delay. In most cases it will turn out to be nothing, but all changes need to be checked as there is a small chance that they could be the first sign of cancer. The sooner this is treated, the greater the prospects of you being helped.

Cervical cancer

What is it ? •

The cervix is the bottom part of the womb (uterus), often called the 'neck'. You can feel it by placing a finger as far back into your vagina as you can. Cancer of the cervix normally takes several years to develop, but, before it does, the cells in the area start to change, providing an early warning system. These changes can be detected if the cells are examined under a microscope. The medical term for the changes is cervical intra-epithelial neoplasia, CIN. The seriousness of the changes is graded from CIN 1 – mild change to CIN 3 – severe changes.

If abnormal cells are not spotted during the early stages of change, they may develop into a tumour, which will require more extensive treatment such as radiation therapy, or surgery, or both.

In most cases of cervical cancer, you will not experience any symptoms, which makes it vitally important to have regular smear tests to detect any pre-cancer changes. If you do experience symptoms such as bleeding between periods, especially after intercourse, bleeding after you have reached the menopause, or a discharge, which may be offensive, you should always check them out with your doctor.

More than 2,000 women in Britain die from cervical cancer each year, and many of these deaths could be prevented through detecting and treating early changes. Sadly, 80 per cent of women who die from cervical cancer have never had a smear test.

Until recent years, cervical cancer affected mainly older women, especially those over 50, but over the last fifteen years there has been an increase among younger women. The cervix in younger women is vulnerable because it is not fully developed, and the increased incidence of cervical cancer in this group may be owing to the earlier age that girls have sexual intercourse. Although overall rates of cervical cancer are falling, the incidence and death rates in younger women in England and Wales is increasing. African-Caribbean women have an increased mortality from cervical cancer; and there is a high incidence in some Asian countries, including India, so that studies are needed to determine whether Asian women living in this country are a high risk group.

The following factors affect your risk of developing cervical cancer

- having first sexual intercourse at a young age – barrier methods of contraception are especially important for young women.
- you are or have been heterosexually active – it's very rare in virgins.
- you smoke – this may double your chances of developing cervical cancer. And if your partner smokes this may also increase your risk to a smaller extent.
- use of the contraceptive pill increases the risk – especially prolonged use (over four years or more); barrier methods of contraception reduce it.
- if you or your partner work in contact with substances like dust, metal, chemicals, machine oil, textiles.
- if you have had several sexual partners, or your partners have had several sexual partners.

- if you or your partner have genital wart virus HPV; barrier methods of contraception can help.
- genital herpes virus may be a risk factor.

It's important not to panic. Even if many of the risk factors apply to you, it doesn't mean you will get cervical cancer. And there are a number of things you can do to reduce your risk.

Make sure you have a smear test once every three years — or more often if you feel you are at particular risk. Abnormal smears are usually followed up at either six-monthly or yearly intervals.

If you are heterosexually active, use a barrier method of contraception, such as the condom, cap or diaphragm, or other safer sex practice (see Contraception, pages 68-70).

Give up smoking (see pages 241-251).

Pay attention to hygiene – you and your partner should wash your sex organs before sex, especially if either of you has a dirty or dusty job.

Follow healthy eating guidelines (see pages 215-228). A high fat diet may be linked with cervical cancer.

The smear test

What is the test?

- A special test (cervical smear test) can detect pre-cancerous changes in the cells of the cervix. Cervical cancer takes many years to develop. The test can show up abnormal cell changes at a stage when they cause no symptoms, when they can be treated easily, and before they develop into a serious condition.

Some changes in cells of the cervix are normal, for example at puberty, during pregnancy or the menopause; others may be a reaction to an infection and will go away when the infection is cleared up. But some may indicate that the cells are developing in a way which may lead to cervical cancer, in which case treatment to prevent this happening will be needed.

Who can have a smear test ?

All women aged 20 to 64 years are now offered a free cervical smear test by the NHS. Depending on where you live, you may be invited every three years or every five. You need to be registered with your GP in order to be invited for a test. You cannot be tested when you are having a period, so make an appointment before or after your period is due.

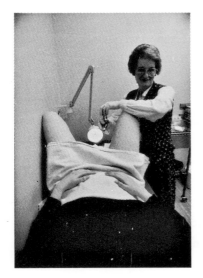

If you have never had a smear test, or have not had one in the last five years, you should go to your doctor or a clinic (see below) and ask for one. You can also ask for one to be done more frequently (at least once a year) if you feel you are at particular risk or are worried about any symptoms. Pre-cancer changes can develop in women of any age. If you have reached the menopause, you still need to be tested; and if you are 65 or over you should ask your doctor how often you need to be screened, though most screening stops at this age, providing you have previously had normal smears.

Where to go for the test

Your own doctor or family planning clinic will give you a smear test; or you may go to a Well-Women (see pages 307-308) or special clinic. Post-natal clinics will usually test you if you have just had a baby. Sometimes it is possible to have a smear test at your workplace (see Health at work, pages 325-327).

What happens at the test

A qualified nurse or doctor will carry out the test, which takes just a few minutes. You will be asked to undress from the waist down and lie on a couch. A small instrument called a speculum will be gently inserted into your vagina to view the cervix. Then a smooth wooden or plastic spatula will be lightly wiped over the inside to pick up a few cells from your cervix. These are put on a slide, and sent away to a laboratory for examination under a microscope. The test may be a little uncomfortable, but is not painful. It will be more comfortable if you can relax – breathing deeply will help.

If you feel embarrassed about having a male doctor carry out the test, you can ask to see a female doctor or nurse when you make your appointment.

Getting the results   •   Make sure you find out when you have the test how and roughly when you will get the result. It usually takes about three weeks. Your doctor may send the result to your home address, or you may be told that you will only be contacted if there is a problem. If you are worried you can always ring and ask for confirmation that your test is all right.

If the smear is positive   •   Try not to panic if you are asked to come back because of the result of a smear test. Only rarely does this mean that you have cancer. It might only be that your sample didn't show up clearly, and another smear is needed. Or it could point to some slight changes in the cells or an infection that can be treated easily. It's important to follow your doctor's advice and have another smear.

If you have an abnormal smear test, you will be asked back to see your doctor or referred directly to a hospital specialist for a colposcopy – a simple, painless examination of the cervix through a high-powered microscope placed at the entrance to your vagina, which shows up the area covered by abnormal cells. As with the smear test, you should not have your period when you have this done. Remember that if you are feeling very anxious, it may help to take your partner or a friend along with you.

The colposcopy will indicate where changes have occurred in the cells of the cervix, and what treatment is recommended. In many cases, the treatment of abnormal cells is quite a minor procedure and, if done early enough, it almost always leads to a complete cure.

Treatment for cervical cancer

If abnormal cells are spotted early enough, one of the following treatments may be recommended. They are simple and almost always lead to a complete cure.

Laser treatment •

If the number of abnormal cells is small, laser treatment may be recommended. A high-energy beam is trained directly on to the abnormal cells to destroy them. You will be given a local anaesthetic, and the treatment doesn't take long, but it may be a little uncomfortable.

Cryocautery •

Gas is used to freeze and destroy the abnormal cells. It takes around ten to fifteen minutes, and you may experience some aching, or a hot, flushing sensation.

Cone biopsy •

This involves the surgical removal of a cone-shaped portion of the cervix, under a general anaesthetic. You will probably need to stay in hospital for a few days. Only the tip of the cervix is removed, and it will not affect your ability to have children.

If cervical cancer has developed beyond the early stages, then more extensive treatment will be needed, either radiation therapy or surgery, or both, depending on all sorts of factors such as your age, general health and the size of the tumour. You should talk to your GP or to your specialist about the best course of treatment.

Skin cancer

What is it ? •

The sun emits some of its energy in the form of ultra-violet light of different wavelengths, certain of which can burn us and cause skin cancer. When you are exposed to strong sun, your skin produces a pigment called melanin to block out the rays and protect the deeper layers of skin. Melanin may take a few days to appear, and is what gives you your tan. If you try to tan faster than your skin can produce melanin, you may risk developing skin cancer. The lighter your skin, the greater the risk.

There are two different types of skin cancer

Non-melanoma

- Non-melanoma skin cancer is more common. Symptoms are small lumps, like warts, which may itch and bleed. They are often found on the head and neck. If detected early they are almost always curable.

Malignant melanoma

- Malignant melanoma can be cured if found early enough and treated quickly. You may notice a change in the normal look of a skin mole. Malignant melanomas grow or change shape. They are often patchy with dark and light areas and may itch and bleed. If you notice any of these symptoms you must see a doctor immediately. They may not be signs of cancer but, if they are, early detection improves your chances of successful treatment.

How common is it ?

- Skin cancer is the second most common cancer in the UK and, while most types are completely curable, some can be fatal. In the UK, melanoma is twice as common in women as in men. For women between the ages of 15 and 64, it is the fourth most common cancer. Women with white skin have little protective melanin pigment, and have an incidence of skin cancer 10 to 12 times higher than black women with the same lifestyle.

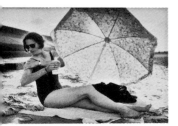

Cases of malignant melanoma have risen rapidly over the last 30 years. This may be because of our changing holiday patterns, as many people now take holidays in countries where the sun is hotter.

How to reduce your risks

- if you want to tan, do it gradually and don't allow yourself to burn.
- only stay in the sun for a short time to begin with.
- use sun lotion to protect you from sunburn and skin cancer. Choose one that has the correct sun protection factor (SPF) for your skin (see below).
- take care even in the shade. Water, sun and snow can reflect sunlight.

Choosing the right lotion

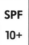

SPF
10+

If you burn easily and tan only with difficulty.

SPF
8+

If you tan easily but sometimes burn.

SPF
6+

If you tan easily.

SPF
2+

If your skin is naturally brown or black.

- treat sun beds with caution. Don't go for a rapid tan, but allow your skin to darken over a period of several weeks. If you are under 16, you burn easily in the sun, or have a family history of skin cancer, sun beds should be avoided.

- don't forget your eyes – wear sunglasses.

- most people have some moles on their skin which remain harmless all their lives. But new, growing or changing moles should be shown to your doctor straightaway.

To guard against sunburn and skin cancer, a sun lotion must filter out the most harmful of the sun's rays. A sun lotion's numerical protection factor is a measure of how well it does this. The higher the SPF, the longer you can stay in the sun without burning. The paler your skin, the higher your recommended SPF.

These SPFs are the lowest for your type of skin. But if you are blond, blue-eyed, red haired or freckled you should choose a lotion with an even higher SPF. These SPFs apply to a warm British summer day. If you're holidaying abroad, the hotter it is, the higher your recommended SPF. If in doubt about which is the right sun lotion for you, ask your pharmacist.

Cardiovascular Disease

Coronary heart disease and stroke both come under the overall heading of cardiovascular disease, and together are second only to all types of cancer as the leading cause of premature death in women in the UK. We have one of the highest rates in the world, with rates in England and Wales about six times that of Japan.

Coronary heart disease

Coronary heart disease (CHD) is used to cover a number of related conditions, including angina, myocardial infarction and sudden

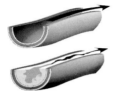

ischaemic death. The most common cause of heart disease is atheroma, a fatty deposit in the arteries, which builds up gradually over time, and may eventually block one or more arteries supplying blood to the heart. If a partial block occurs, it may cause chest pain, known as angina. If the block is complete, part of the heart dies from lack of oxygen and other nutrients, leading to a heart attack (known as a coronary thrombosis or myocardial infarction).

Stroke

Stroke may be caused when atheroma (the fatty deposits) leads to a narrowing of blood vessels supplying the brain. It is directly related to high blood pressure, which becomes more common as you get older. 10 per cent of strokes are caused by bleeding from weak areas in the brain's blood vessels, which is also directly linked to high blood pressure.

Who is at risk?

Women get heart disease too

- Heart disease is the leading single cause of death in the UK, and we have one of the highest rates in the world. Many people think of men, not women, as suffering from heart disease and getting heart attacks, and most research has been carried out on men. Although overall women suffer fewer heart attacks than men, they have the same rates of angina, and coronary heart disease is the single greatest cause of death in women both above and below the age of 65. Little has been explored about what protects women from heart disease compared with men. Both the positive and negative aspects of our lives may be a clue to developing a more effective approach to preventing CHD.

Which women?

- The incidence of heart disease is strongly linked with social class, even after the classic risk factors (see pages 183-186) have been taken into account, with working-class women having a higher incidence than professional women. The sort of job we do affects our risk of coronary heart disease. A study on civil servants found that those in the lowest grade, poorly paid jobs had nearly four times the death rate from heart disease as those in the highest, best-paid jobs. The workers worst affected also experienced social isolation, having little contact with workmates, friends or family. Although only men were included in this study, it is not difficult to extrapolate the results to women, many of whom are in routine jobs with little or no control over their work, outside or inside the home, with little money, and who often feel isolated and trapped. A study on women, based in America, found that those with children, doing low-paid repetitive and routine jobs were twice as likely to get heart disease as women who worked in their homes. These factors may be just as useful at predicting who will get heart disease as the more accepted risk factors such as smoking, blood pressure and high cholesterol levels.

Women from certain minority ethnic groups are also at greater risk of heart disease and stroke. Between 1979 and 1983, death from coronary heart disease was 46 per cent higher among women who had been born in the Indian subcontinent than the national average, with the risk being greatest among the young. Women from the Caribbean have a low incidence of heart disease, though they are at much greater risk of stroke, with about double the national average. Those from the Indian subcontinent and the African Commonwealth are also more likely to die from a stroke.

One theory, the 'Type A Theory', has suggested that different types of personality make you more or less prone to heart disease. The person who finds it hard to relax, is always pressed for time, is competitive and aggressive, is thought to be at greater risk than someone who is calm, less competitive and more relaxed.

Traditionally, women who have a male partner take on themselves the responsibility for keeping him healthy and, in particular, protecting him from heart disease. They also adopt responsibility for the general well-being of the rest of the family. Health promotion messages are quick to point to women to make sure that they choose and prepare healthy foods, help their partner relax, encourage them to be active, and generally ensure that the family lifestyle is such that there will be minimum risk of heart disease. These messages often fail to point out to women that they themselves are also at risk. Women may find it particularly difficult to take preventive action for themselves, because of the day-to-day stress of coping with work and family responsibilities, and because they tend to put their own needs last.

How can you reduce your risk?

CHD is caused by a combination of factors. There is no way of changing some of the risk factors such as your family history of heart disease, or your age. But other risks include smoking, high blood pressure, high blood cholesterol levels, being overweight, being physically inactive, and high alcohol consumption, and these can be reduced by making personal changes. There is some evidence to suggest that stress may also contribute to your chances of developing heart disease, but this association is not fully understood at the moment. When several risk factors occur together, they combine to cause a considerable increase in the risk of a heart attack.

Smoking • Smoking is a major risk factor – for more information see pages 238-241.

Being active • Most of us work hard, but at sedentary jobs or work around the home. Neither raises our pulse rate nor builds up a sweat. The heart is the one muscle of the body which never stops working, and it needs exercise more than any other. You should exercise regularly at least three times a week and for around twenty minutes each time – it doesn't have to be a sport – anything which gets you out of breath and moving faster will be a benefit (see Activity, pages 196-197).

Aspirin • A recent major trial in the British Medical Journal suggests that a significant reduction in mortality from strokes and heart disease could be achieved by a daily low dose of aspirin for those at high risk.

Blood cholesterol •

The risk of CHD rises progressively with increasing concentrations of blood cholesterol. Average blood cholesterol levels in the UK are high by international standards. Among men and women aged between 18 and 64 they are 5.8 mmol/l, compared with the recommended cut-off point of 5.2 mmol/l for adult men (although this should perhaps be higher for women). There has been little change in levels over the last twenty years. The typical diet in the UK is too high in saturated fat, sugars and cholesterol. When taken in excess, these can cause fatty deposits (atheroma) to build up in the lining of major arteries. In the same way that pipes may clog up with limescale, the arteries may gradually become narrower, obstructing the blood flow and making the heart work harder.

In pre-menopausal women, circulating levels of the hormone oestrogen may help to protect us from CHD by keeping levels of blood cholesterol down. And we may also be protected by substances called high-density lipoproteins (HDL). After the menopause, natural levels of oestrogen fall and there is a corresponding increase in incidence of CHD. Blood cholesterol levels among women increase with age, and from about the age of 50 are higher than in men. By the age of 55, over 75 per cent of women have levels above 6.5 mmol/l, and nearly a third of them have levels over 7.8 mmol/l. However, cholesterol levels may be less important for women, and for any given level of cholesterol, women have roughly a third the risk of men of developing coronary heart disease in the next six years. This may be because of our relatively low triglyceride and high HDL cholesterol levels. There is no conclusive research about the benefits of reducing blood cholesterol levels in women, so that the best course of treatment is, as yet, unclear.

A number of factors affect blood cholesterol levels – diet, the contraceptive pill, how active you are:

Diet •   Diet plays an important part. Diets containing a lot of fat, and particularly saturated fats, can cause high levels of blood cholesterol. While the expert government committee on food (COMA) recommends the amount of fat we eat should not exceed 35 per cent of our food energy intake, a recent survey has found that only 15 per cent of women achieve this target at present. Even more worrying, fewer than 3 per cent of women are at or below the recommended level for saturated fat (which is 11 per cent food energy). Over the last 20 years, the amount of saturated fat in our diet has gone down, in particular because we are eating less butter, full fat milk and red meat. But there has been an increase in the amount of hidden fat we eat in foods like biscuits, chocolate and ice-cream, meaning that overall we still eat too much saturated fat. Cutting down on fat in our diet in general will help. There is also some evidence that eating lots of soluble fibre, such as oats and pulses, may help to reduce blood cholesterol levels.

The pill •   The oral contraceptive pill has a marked effect on levels of hormones and other substances in the body, thus increasing the risk of heart disease amongst users. Women who smoke and take the pill have 40 times the risk of a heart attack and 22 times the risk of stroke compared with women on the pill who do not smoke.

Predisposition •   Familial hypercholesterolaemia is an inherited disorder affecting about one person in 500, and causing abnormally high levels of blood cholesterol and a high risk of premature death from CHD.

Physical activity •   Physical activity helps to lower total levels of blood cholesterol, and may help raise high density lipoproteins (HDL) which remove cholesterol deposited in arterial walls, thereby reducing the risk of heart disease.

Cholesterol testing – •   There is debate at present about the value of cholesterol testing, and it is
pros and cons   generally agreed that it should be offered only to individuals with an increased risk of CHD, as part of an overall CHD prevention programme.

There is some doubt at present about the importance of cholesterol as a risk factor for coronary heart disease in women. Blood cholesterol levels should only be assessed in the context of overall coronary heart disease risk assessment, taking other factors into account. It may be appropriate for you if you have:

- a close relative under the age of 50 with myocardial infarction
- a family history or clinical signs of high levels of blood lipids (hyperlipidaemias)
- a personal history of diabetes, or CHD under age 65

or with two or more of the following risk factors:

- smoking
- hypertension
- obesity
- inadequate physical activity levels.

The blood cholesterol level at which therapy, such as diet or drug treatment, is recommended is higher in women than in men. A number of commercial outlets, pharmacies, and screening services may offer cholesterol testing. If you decide to have your cholesterol level measured in this way, and are concerned or unsure about the result, you should talk to your doctor.

Blood pressure

Around a fifth of women in the UK develop high blood pressure, known as hypertension, at some time in their lives. Blood pressure tends to rise naturally with age, and after the age of 45 women's average blood pressure is higher than men's. Many people with high blood pressure experience no symptoms, so that it may go untreated for some time. Severe cases may have warning signs such as bad headaches, dizziness or fainting. High blood pressure can cause stroke, may led to heart disease and can cause problems with the eyes, kidneys, brain, and during pregnancy.

Blood pressure and the oral contraceptive pill

Many women on the combined oral contraceptive pill (oestrogen and progestogen combined) get a slight increase in blood pressure. A few will develop high blood pressure, and the longer you use the pill the more likely this is. You should have your blood pressure checked before starting to use the pill, and then regularly thereafter. If you are overweight, or have a family history of hypertension, you should keep a particularly careful check on your blood pressure.

Blood pressure in different ethnic groups

African-Caribbean women have an increased risk of high blood pressure. The incidence of stroke and death from hypertensive disease in England and Wales between 1979 and 1983 was seven times greater in Caribbean women than the national average. Asian women and women from the African Commonwealth also have a higher incidence of high blood pressure, though not as marked as for Caribbeans.

Preventing or reducing hypertension

There are a number of things you can do to prevent high blood pressure, or to reduce it.

Giving up smoking • Giving up smoking is probably the single most important way to control your blood pressure (see Smoking, pages 236-251).

Regular physical activity • Regular physical activity can help your heart to work more efficiently, and can help to reduce blood pressure (see Physical activity, pages 194-197).

If you already suffer from blood pressure, you should talk to your doctor and agree a sensible exercise programme. If you experience any dizzy spells, headaches or sudden pain when you are exercising, keep moving and ease down gently.

Reducing salt intake • Reducing salt intake may help prevent or treat high blood pressure (see Healthy eating, pages 215-217). The easiest way to do this is to stop using salt in cooking and at the table, and cut down on processed foods which provide around three-quarters of the salt in our diet.

Avoiding being overweight • Avoiding being overweight can help, especially together with exercise (see Weight control, page 228).

Sensible drinking • Sensible drinking can help. If you take more than the recommended 14 units of alcohol per week, you have a greater risk of raised blood pressure. Drinking can also contribute to obesity.

HRT and heart disease

Oestrogen therapy has been shown to reduce the risk of CHD in post-menopausal women by up to 50 per cent. However, the preparations more widely prescribed today contain a combination of oestrogen and progrestogen, and these may have less benefit. At present there is insufficient evidence to conclude whether the benefits of combined hormone replacement therapy for cardiovascular risk outweigh the risks of increased breast cancer.

If you are thinking about taking HRT or are already using it, you need to talk through the pros and cons with your doctor.

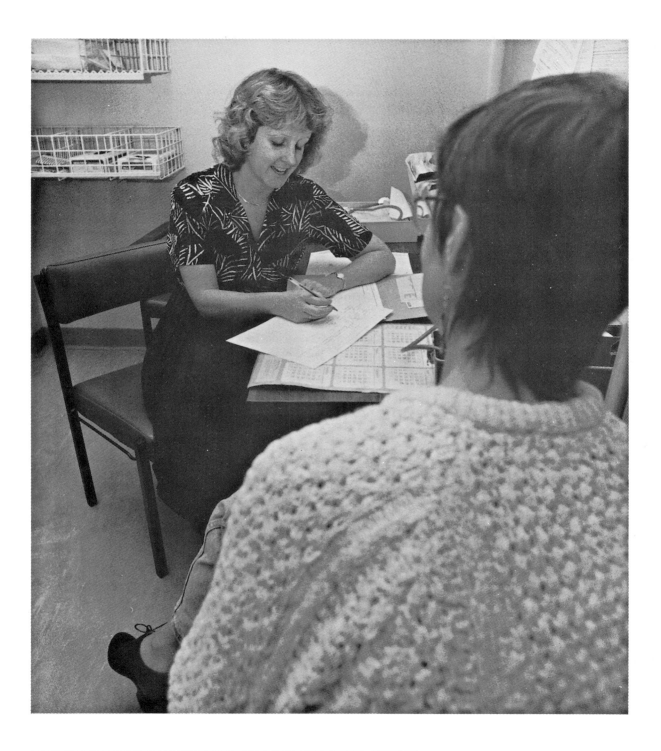

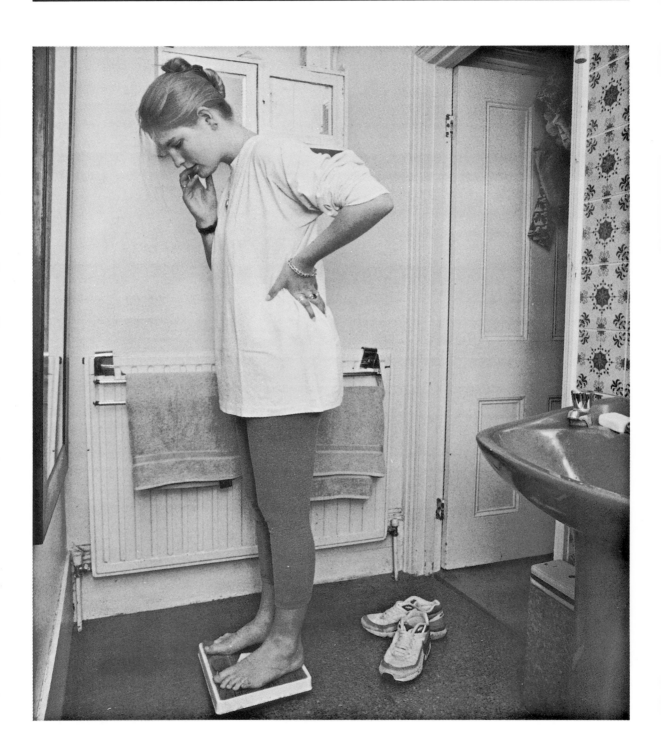

What Makes Us Healthy?

To a great extent what makes us healthy or unhealthy is how we live our lives day to day – whether we get enough rest, relaxation, and physical activity; what we eat; whether we smoke or use other drugs; how much alcohol we use; how safe our workplace is; and how much stress we have. It's about our relationships too – whether there are people we can trust and confide in; and friends we can enjoy ourselves with.

You know that there are certain changes you could make to improve your health. But there are many reasons why women find it hard to follow good advice and build healthy practices into their lives. Work and family responsibilities put pressures on us, leaving us rushing round trying to fit everything in, to make sure everyone else is taken care of while neglecting our own needs.

Many of the factors affecting our health are beyond our control. Lack of money, where you live, the work you do, too much to do with not enough support, environmental problems, all have an impact on our health, and you may feel unable to do much about them. If your life is full of the stress of coping with children, holding down a job and making ends meet, how do you find the time or energy to relax or exercise? And how can you choose the lean cuts of meat and plenty of fruit and vegetables if you're on a tight budget? It's too simplistic to blame individuals for the way they live without taking into account some of the reasons behind those decisions.

It's not always easy to change. Patterns and habits build up gradually over long periods of time. It feels comfortable to do the things you've always done, and trying something new may feel risky. There's also pressure from those around you. Children may complain bitterly if you decide to make even the smallest changes to the contents of the fridge; your partner may be equally resistant to any suggestions you make;

friends may accuse you of being a damp squib when you say you're looking after your health.

This chapter helps you consider where you could make changes to improve or protect your health, to think about what might be stopping you from achieving this, and to plan how to go about it. Be realistic about what you can achieve and take things one step at a time. Begin with small changes that you can make right now, rather than large-scale plans, such as getting a new job or finding a different relationship, which might take rather longer. You can work towards those more challenging goals while getting a sense of achievement and feeling the benefit from the smaller changes you make. Go easy on yourself and try not to let getting healthy become yet another area of your life which rules you and leaves you feeling a failure. Make it something you do for yourself, giving you a feeling of choice and power, and leaving you feeling good.

Being Active

Why be active?

There is growing evidence that regular physical activity is good for our health. A recent report from the Royal College of Physicians showed it to be effective in improving circulation and reducing your chances of coronary heart disease; strengthening muscles and bones (especially important for women in helping to prevent the onset of osteoporosis); helping to control your weight; improving suppleness and stamina and protecting against back problems. Being active can make you better able to resist infections and, if you do fall ill, you're likely to recover much more quickly. It will help you cope with stress, too, protect against depression, and improve your self-esteem. It can even improve your sex life.

A major national fitness survey published by the Sports Council and Health Education Authority in 1992 found that eight out of ten women fall below the level of activity needed to benefit their health. This is true for women of all ages, and the older women get, the less active they are.

Life used to be so physically demanding that it was unheard of to spend time especially for exercising. But things have changed. Despite the stresses of living and working today, few of us do the kind of work or have a lifestyle which gives us enough activity. Life in the 1990s is dominated by machines – those of us fortunate enough to have cars drive the smallest distance rather than walk, in the interest of saving time; household tasks have been revolutionised (thank goodness!) to remove the drudgery but also the physical labour; and leisure time is dominated by sedentary pastimes such as watching television and eating. Be honest! You probably aren't as active or fit as you think. Most of us would benefit from doing more – the important thing is to choose activities that you can easily fit into your day-to-day life, so that you enjoy them and keep going.

What is fitness?

Fitness is to do with having suppleness, strength and stamina:

Suppleness • Being able to bend, stretch, twist and turn through a full range of movements. You need it all the time – for awkward jobs around the house, getting in and out of cars and on to buses and trains. If you're supple, you're less likely to get injured and you'll be able to stay more active as you get older.

Strength • Being able to exert force – for pushing, pulling and lifting. You need strength all the time – to move around, carry shopping or children, climb stairs. It protects you from sprains and strains. A strong back and tummy will help give you a good posture too.

Stamina • Being able to keep going, when running or walking briskly, without getting tired and puffed very quickly. Stamina is useful when you're in a hurry to get somewhere, or when you need to keep up with your children! Exercising for stamina helps protect you against heart disease.

The best activities for stamina are fairly energetic (more than you are used to), make you slightly out of breath and keep you moving for twenty minutes or more. This type of exercise is often called 'aerobic' exercise because you breathe in enough oxygen to supply your working muscles.

How fit are you?

If you answer yes to any of the following you would benefit from being more active.

Do you quickly get out of breath walking uphill or even on the flat?	**Yes** — You need to improve your stamina. Walking more is the best way to start.	**No** — Good. If you want to build up even more stamina, try swimming or cycling.
Do your legs ache or feel weak after you've climbed a couple of flights of stairs?	**Yes** — You need more leg strength.	**No** — Good. Your legs are fairly strong. If you want them to get even stronger you could cycle or jog.
Do you find it difficult to bend down and tie your shoelaces, or put your socks or tights on?	**Yes** — You need to improve your suppleness.	**No** — You're reasonably supple. It's worth making the effort to keep it that way as you get older.
Do you find it difficult to comb the back of your hair or pull a jumper off?	**Yes** — You need more flexibility in your shoulder joints.	**No** — Good. Keep moving.
Is it difficult for you to get out of an armchair or the bath?	**Yes** — You need to improve your suppleness, and the strength in your arms and legs.	**No** — Good. You'll find it a great advantage to work on your strength and suppleness, especially as you get older.

Many health centres, clubs and gyms offer more elaborate tests of stamina, suppleness and strength to give you an overall fitness rating.

What sort of activity?

There are many different types of physical activity, and all can make a useful contribution to your overall level of fitness. Sports provide the opportunity for some of the most vigorous activity, and there are literally hundreds of different ones to choose from, to suit all levels of ability and fitness. Exercise and leisure pursuits are another good way to keep active. Physical activity is also part of everyday life – climbing stairs, carrying shopping, getting to and from work, looking after children or an elderly relative can be very physically demanding. But even if you're pretty active at home or work, you'll probably still need other activities to give you enough suppleness, stamina and strength.

The most important thing is that you ENJOY it. It's not following some gruelling work-out or putting yourself through an endurance test. If you go down that road you know you'll never stick to it anyway. Rather than think of it just as a means to an end, take time to choose something you will enjoy and that will make you feel good.

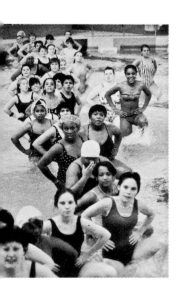

There's certainly no shortage of different sorts of activities to suit all levels of ability and fitness. If you're the sporty type, then anything from badminton or basketball to fencing or ice-hockey may fit the bill. If not, you may want to think about activities involving movement such as dance, yoga or keep fit. If the social side is important, join a class, or gym if you can afford it. If you prefer to exercise alone, then cycling, swimming or walking may be good choices. You don't have to stick to traditional sports and exercise activities – jiving can be just as good for you as jogging, and gardening may do you as much good as a friendly game of tennis.

Don't be too complacent about how much exercise you're getting. Your conscience may prompt you into going along to a class every week, or jogging on a Sunday morning. But although you're doing better than the stay-at-homes, it's still not enough to make a real difference. All the evidence shows that while it doesn't have to hurt, to benefit your health you need to:

• do something energetic which gets you out of breath and sweaty for twenty minutes, three times a week

- spend half-an-hour or more each day doing things that make your heart beat a bit faster – climbing stairs, walking, digging the garden or dancing are all good.

This may sound rather daunting and unrealistic. The key is to try to make the most of everyday opportunities that offer the chance to exert yourself – walk up stairs and escalators rather than riding or taking the lift; walk whenever you can – to the shops, all or part of the way to work; do more strenuous activities around the house and garden; and make time for some regular energetic pursuits that you enjoy.

Spoilt for choice!

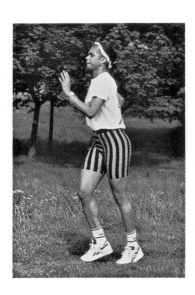

There have never been more opportunities and choices when it comes to physical activity. **Walking** is the most natural exercise of all. Brisk walking is great for stamina, but for all-round fitness it's best to take some other form of exercise as well. **Swimming** is excellent for strength, stamina and suppleness, especially if you use various strokes. It's a great way to get fit and stay fit, especially if you're overweight or have backache, stiffness or a disability, because your body is supported by water. **Cycling** is very good for stamina and leg strength. It won't do much for suppleness if you're young, but as you get older it really helps to keep you moving. **Jogging** and **running** at an easy pace is very popular. It's fun, free and a quick way to get fit. It's very good for stamina, but not so good for suppleness or upper body strength. Be careful not to overdo it at first – run on soft surfaces like grass when you can. If you have arthritis in your legs, hips or back or are overweight, try swimming or cycling instead. **Bowling** is not too energetic and improves flexibility in shoulders and arms, and strength in legs. **Badminton** is fun even if you're a beginner. It involves lots of bending, stretching and leaping, so it's good for flexibility and strength, especially leg strength. You're moving all the time so it also helps stamina. **Tennis** is good for stamina, pretty good for suppleness, and certainly good for leg strength, and the

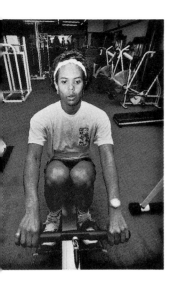

exercise value gets better as your game improves. For squash you have to be fit, so don't play **squash** to get fit. It can be excellent for stamina, leg strength and suppleness. If you're middle-aged, think carefully before taking it up and, if you do decide to play, take it very gently at first. **Team games** are also good for stamina and strength, and pretty good for suppleness. You don't have to play seriously – you can play for fun on the beach or at the park. **Weight training** is becoming more and more popular, especially with women. Whether you train with free weights or machines, you will become stronger and build up stamina. Suitable training can firm up your body and help you become slim and supple. You need to learn the proper techniques for lifting, or you risk damaging your knees, shoulders and back, or straining yourself. **Martial arts** and **judo** involve physical workout, relaxation and skill-learning. They are good for stamina, suppleness and strength. **Exercise classes** cover aerobics, circuit training, exercise to music, keep fit, and over-60s classes, and many others. An all-over work-out is good for stamina, strength and suppleness. Some exercises build up strength in your legs, arms, tummy and back. Gentle bending and stretching is good for suppleness. And aerobic exercises are great for stamina. **Dancing** is getting more and more popular, and whatever the type, you're getting really good exercise. The more energetically you dance, the better it is for your stamina. It keeps your joints supple and mobile. It's good for balance, too, and that's important as you get older. **Yoga** is great for suppleness and general relaxation because it's gentle and controlled. It's good for strengthening muscles, especially in the stomach, hips, thighs and back, although there's very little benefit for stamina.

Exercising at home

Lots of people prefer to exercise at home. Exercising at home has distinct advantages. It's private and there's no need to get a babysitter or travel anywhere. You might get more out of it if you go to a class first and learn how to do it properly.

Exercising for suppleness

These six simple stretching exercises should be done at least three times a week – you'll feel your body becoming more supple and relaxed. You should also do them to warm up before starting anything more vigorous.

Do all stretching exercises slowly and smoothly. Repeat each one eight to twelve times. Do a few the first day and gradually build up. If you have trouble with back pain, it may be sensible to see a doctor first.

Arm circling •   To maintain suppleness in your shoulders. Stand tall and relaxed with your arms at your sides. Slowly circle your right shoulder backwards. Repeat with your left shoulder and continue on alternate sides.

Place your right hand on your right shoulder. Move your elbow forwards, up, and back, in a circle. Repeat with your left elbow, and continue on both sides. Start with your arms straight at your sides. Keep your hips facing forward and move your right arm forward, up, and back, to form a large circle. Repeat on the left and continue on alternate sides.

Any of these arm circles can be done with both arms together.

Forward bending •   To stretch the muscles in your shoulders, trunk and legs. Stand tall and relaxed. Stretching through your whole body, reach towards the ceiling with your fingertips. Then, letting yourself bend at the hips and knees, slowly bring your hands down towards the floor, as far as is comfortable. Straighten up and repeat.

Side bending •   To stretch the muscles in your sides and help keep your spine flexible. Stand tall and relaxed with your feet apart and hands at your sides. Slowly bend to the left and right alternately, allowing your hands to slide down the sides of your legs. Stand tall between bends. Keep your legs straight. Make sure you are bending to the side and not letting your

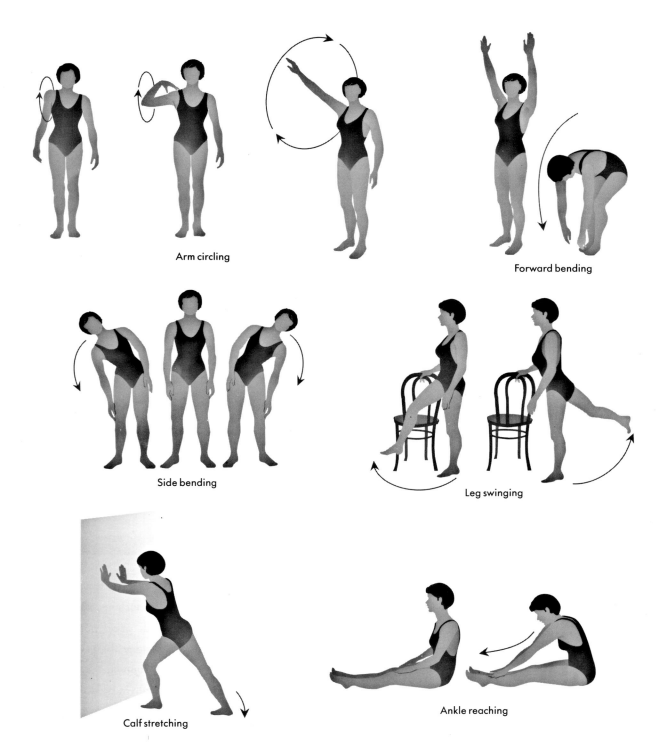

Arm circling

Forward bending

Side bending

Leg swinging

Calf stretching

Ankle reaching

shoulders drop forwards. Move only as far as you can comfortably and return to the upright position. Don't bounce into the movement.

Leg swinging • To keep your hips mobile and to stretch the thigh muscles. Stand tall and relaxed with your weight on your left leg. Rest your left hand on the back of a chair for support, if necessary. Now swing your right leg forwards and backwards in a relaxed, pendulum action. Gradually take your leg as high as you comfortably can, keeping your body fairly upright and letting your right knee bend. Repeat with your left leg.

Calf stretching • To stretch your calves and keep your ankles mobile. Stand facing a wall, at arm's length from it. Place your hands on the wall for support and stretch your right leg out straight behind you with the ball of your foot on the floor and your toes pointing towards the wall. Gently push your right heel towards the floor, allowing your left leg to bend as necessary (but no further than is shown in the picture).

Ankle reaching • To stretch your lower back and the backs of your thighs. Sit on the floor with your legs straight out in front of you and your knees as near to the floor as is comfortable. Place your hands on top of your thighs. Slowly and smoothly slide your hands down your legs as far as you can comfortably reach. Return to the upright position and repeat. Do not bounce into the movement.

Exercising for strength

It helps to keep your muscles toned up enough to meet the strenuous demands of daily life. You need strong arms for pushing, pulling and lifting. Strong stomach muscles are important for good posture and avoiding back pain. You need strong legs for many things including getting out of chairs and baths, climbing stairs and running. It's especially important for older people to maintain their strength in order to remain active and independent. Try these exercises every day, or at least twice a week. Don't push yourself too hard to start with. Five or six repeats will probably be plenty to start with. Build up gently and gradually to twenty repeats. You will find that it soon becomes easier and enjoyable.

Arms   1   To strengthen mostly upper arms, shoulders and chest.

Wall press-up   •   Stand at arm's length from a wall. Place your hands shoulder-width apart on the wall. Now bend your arms until your forehead touches the wall. Then push yourself away again until your arms are straight.

Kneeling press-up   •   Kneel on all fours. Move your hands forward slightly and take most of your weight on to them. Bend your arms and lower the top half of your body towards the floor. Only go as far as is comfortable, and be careful not to sag in the middle. Straighten your arms again and return to the starting position.

Full press-up   •   If you can do the kneeling press-ups easily you may be ready to attempt a full press-up. Follow the instructions above but alter the starting position by lifting your knees off the floor, so that your weight is supported on your hands and toes and your body is in a straight line.

Stomach, back and hips   2   To help strengthen your stomach muscles, flatten any bulges and improve your posture.

Curl ups   •   To strengthen your tummy muscles.
Lie on your back with your knees bent. Put your hands on the top of your thighs. Lifting just your head and shoulders off the floor, slide your fingers along your thighs as far as is comfortable. Then uncurl slowly back to the lying position.

As an alternative you can do this exercise lying on your back with your feet and lower legs on the seat of a chair.

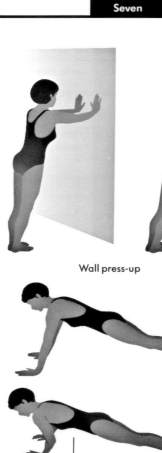

Wall press-up

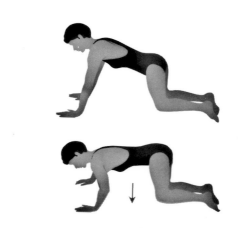

Kneeling press-up

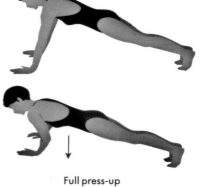

Full press-up

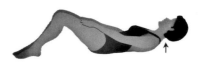
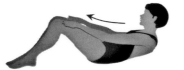

Curl-ups

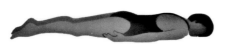

Chest raises

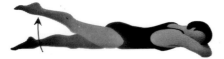

Leg-lifts

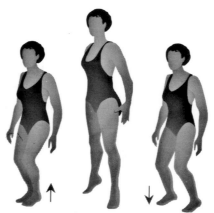

Spring-ups

| Chest raises | • | to strengthen the muscles in your back. Lie on your stomach on the floor, with your arms at your sides, your shoulders relaxed, and your head on one side. Slowly lift your head, neck and shoulders away from the floor, turning your head so you are looking at the floor with your chin tucked in. Only go as far as is comfortable. Slowly relax down turning your head to the other side, and repeat. |

| Leg-lifts | • | to strengthen your hips and back. Lie on your stomach on the floor. Slowly lift your right leg away from the floor, as far as is comfortable. Slowly relax down and repeat with the other leg. |

| Legs | 3 | These will help you tone up and strengthen your thighs, calves and bottom. They are particularly important for older people. |

| Stand-ups | • | Sit on a firm chair. Stand up without using your hands and without leaning forward too much, if you can. Make sure your legs straighten completely. Sit down again and repeat. Gradually progress just to touching the chair instead of sitting down each time. |

| Step-ups | • | Stand at the bottom of a flight of stairs. Step up on to the first step, making sure you straighten both legs. Step down again. Do this with alternate legs. |

| Spring-ups | • | Stand with your feet together and your knees slightly bent. Spring up, landing with your feet comfortably apart and your knees bent. Now spring up again, landing with your feet together. Repeat as a continuous movement – apart, together, apart, together. Once you can do about twenty repeats this exercise will also build your stamina. |

So why don't we do it?

All the recent research points to the fact that as a nation our activity levels are well below those necessary to improve personal health and fitness.

Nearly everyone can benefit from being more active.

Lack of time is a common reason which women give for not getting more physical activity. It's easy to mistake the exhaustion you feel at the end of the day for a sign that you've got all the activity you need; but it's more likely thanks to stress and hassle – and that won't do you any good!

Many of us are put off because we don't see ourselves as sporty. Negative experiences at school leave many of us feeling that we're no good at sport or exercise and that they have nothing to offer in terms of enjoyment or as a sense of achievement. Being overweight puts us off too – it's easy to be alienated by the 'fit and healthy' stereotype of slim young bodies in glamorous leotards, and to feel embarrassed. It may be a tight budget that stops you joining the local aerobics class or visiting the swimming-pool as often as you'd like. But the fact is that being active doesn't have to cost money – you can exercise at home on your own or with friends.

Many women with young children find it hard to make time to indulge in their own activities. Lack of childcare facilities may be a problem. Sports and leisure centres are recognising the needs of mothers, and many now provide crèche facilities – sometimes subsidised or free. One way round the problem of what to do with the children is to find activities you can do together. This becomes a more realistic proposition as children get older. Mother and toddler swimming sessions may give you little chance to swim yourself, unless you go with a friend and take it in turns to watch the children; but once the children can swim competently themselves, a family trip to the pool can be a good chance for some exercise for you. Setting a good example to your children and encouraging them to get into the habit of being active is one of the best things you can do for them. There are lots more family activities that can be fun and keep you all active – walking, cycling, 10-pin bowling, orienteering – the list is virtually endless and there's certainly something for every taste.

If none of this applies to you, then maybe you're shy, or just lack the energy or motivation to get going. Feeling tired may stop you from being active, but the reality is that physical activity can actually leave you feeling refreshed and energetic.

If you want to find ways to get yourself going, some of these suggestions may help:

'I haven't got time. My life is too busy.'

Try fitting some activity into your day – before, between or after other commitments. You could do something with a friend in your lunch break at work, take advantage of uncrowded leisure facilities during the week, once you've dropped the children at school, or combine something active with socialising during the evening. Just twenty minutes, two or three times a week can keep you feeling fit and active.

'I'm not the sporty type.'

Even if you didn't like sport at school, there are now so many different activities you are sure to be able to find one you enjoy. Don't let embarrassment put you off. People of all shapes and sizes enjoy exercising and you won't feel uncomfortable or out of place if you choose an activity that's right for you.

'I've got young children to look after.'

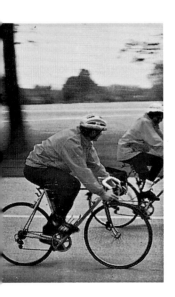

It might take a bit more organising but it doesn't have to stop you exercising. Some sports and leisure centres have childcare facilities (your local library or Leisure and Recreation Department of your Local Authority should be able to tell you about facilities). You could get together with a group of other women with young children to share babysitting.

'I couldn't do it on my own.'

Make the most of local facilities – join one of the many groups or classes on offer, or get together with some friends and go along together.

'What I need is relaxation.'

Exercise can be just the thing to help you relax. It relieves stress by taking your mind off your problems. After vigorous exercise, you'll feel warm, comfortable and relaxed. Exercise can also lift depression, and you'll probably find it helps you sleep better too.

Getting started

Getting started is the hardest step, but once you start to feel the benefits you won't want to give up. Maybe you have spurts of being active from time to time – when you decide you need to lose weight, feel guilty about neglecting your health, or get swept into making a new year's resolution. But other aspects of life take precedence, self-discipline can so easily go out of the window, and because you're not enjoying it you give up.

If you are only just beginning to take regular exercise, you should let your body adjust gradually to the new routine. Of course there may be some aches at first as long-forgotten muscles are rediscovered. But beware of any pain as this is a sign that you are overdoing it. Choose an activity where you can set the pace – if you break yourself in gently, you will quickly begin to feel the benefits, giving an added boost to your willpower to keep going. Always warm up first, with a few gentle bends and stretches. And cool down afterwards by walking slowly for a few minutes. Most injuries are caused by overuse of joints and muscles, so don't overdo it. In general, don't do anything vigorous unless you've worked up to it and you're doing it regularly.

Sensible precautions

Most people, including older people, don't need a medical check-up before starting regular exercise, but ask your doctor about the best form of exercise for you if:

- you've had chest pains, high blood pressure or heart disease.
- you have chest trouble, like asthma or bronchitis.
- you have back trouble or have a slipped disc.
- you're troubled with joint pains or arthritis.
- you have diabetes.
- you're recovering from an illness or operation.
- you're worried that exercise may affect any other aspect of your health.

In all these conditions exercise can be helpful but it's a good idea to talk it over with your doctor first. If in doubt about your health, check with your doctor to plan a personal exercise programme.

Stop exercising if you experience any pain, dizziness, feel sick or unwell, or unusual fatigue. If the symptoms persist or come back later, or if you are worried about them, see your doctor.

Exercise is for everyone

If you're overweight

Increasing your level of activity is an important part of controlling or losing weight. It's not just about toning up – exercise actually uses energy (calories) and raises the metabolic rate, leading to weight loss. There's evidence that some people may still be burning up more calories than usual after they've finished exercising – sometimes for up to 24 hours.

Sometimes, women who are overweight feel embarrassed about

exposing their bodies, lack confidence or feel that exercise sessions are not for people like them. Also, they may worry that physical exertion will do more harm than good. But in fact, they are just the ones who will benefit most from some regular physical activity, especially if it's the stamina-building type.

If you have a disability

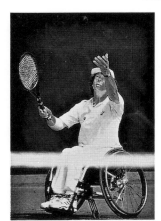

Having a disability doesn't mean you shouldn't exercise. You have just as much to gain from regular activity as anyone else. The barriers you may encounter are often more to do with other people's idea of what is right or safe for you. But many people with disability are now demonstrating just how much they can gain from participating in sport and exercise, and how much they have to offer.

'Being partially sighted, I was very nervous of water but my family gave me lots of encouragement to learn to swim. It took a lot of determination, but now I belong to the local swimming club and swim several times a week.'

When you're pregnant

The general benefits of being active apply just as much during pregnancy as at any other time. Exercise can build up your strength and suppleness so you are better able to cope with the demands on your body during pregnancy, and while you are in labour. It may also help you to relax and sleep better, ensuring you get much-needed rest.

If you're not used to exercising, go gently. It's not the right time to try strenuous new activities. Even if you are very active, sports like skiing and riding are probably best avoided. The best sorts of exercise include swimming, walking, dance and yoga. You shouldn't allow yourself to get tired out – spend shorter periods with plenty of breaks, and relax afterwards to allow your body to recover. You can continue with regular, gentle exercise through most of your pregnancy, easing off in the last few weeks.

As you get older

Keeping active is a positive health benefit for young and old alike. Exercise can fend off many of the difficulties we associate with growing older, keeping us more supple, mobile and independent. The Allied Dunbar National Fitness Survey found a clear association between past participation in sport and physical activity and a lower prevalence of heart disease, angina and breathlessness. Among those who had not taken part in regular activity as adults, 15 per cent of women over 55 suffered from one of these chronic conditions compared with only 3 per cent who had regularly participated for over three-quarters of their adult life.

If you haven't been used to taking part in physical activity, it's never too late to start. You may be worried about not being fit enough for anything energetic, or about overdoing things, but don't underestimate what your body can do. Muscles under-used through a lifetime of neglect will soon firm up with a gentle work-out. Active bodies go hand in hand with active minds. Don't avoid activity because it makes you breathless. It's important not to get into a negative spiral of inactivity – where reduced activity leads to reduced capabilities, which in turn lead to a further reduction in activity.

Build up your activity gradually. Choose something which will stimulate the circulation, keep joints mobile and muscles trim. If the social side is important too, there are lots of groups or classes to join for activities such as dancing, bowls or rambling. Other active interests can be done alone or with friends – swimming or walking, or keep fit at home.

One of the long-term benefits of exercise is the prevention of osteoporosis, or brittle bones, which one woman in four suffers from.

Weight-bearing exercise such as walking, cycling or tennis can significantly reduce the loss of bone that commonly occurs in women as they age. A study in the USA found that bone density in the spine in active women aged 55 to 75 was 15 per cent to 20 per cent greater than in sedentary women of the same age.

Feeling the benefit

More and more women are enjoying sports and exercise. Over the last twenty years, the fitness boom and our increasing awareness of how much good exercise does us has spurred lots of women into taking action. There has been an increase in the facilities available and many sports centres now offer women-only sessions, often with a crèche. You may not be so well provided for if you live in a rural area – it's worth enquiring what your council or local sports centre offers, and if they don't provide what you want at present, ask for it!

Checking your progress

Once you've started exercising regularly, you may find it encouraging to 'test' your fitness to see how much you've improved. Think about whether you can exercise longer now than when you started. When you finish a session of exercise do you feel you could easily do some more?

A simple stamina test

If you've been exercising regularly for at least two months and you want to start keeping a record of your progress, try this test. Don't forget that stamina is only one aspect of fitness. To get really fit, you need to develop your strength and suppleness as well.

- Find a safe, reasonably flat route about one mile long. It could be in a park, on a quiet stretch of road, on a running track, or between your home and a nearby landmark. You can measure the distance with a car mileometer or by using a map.

- Put on comfortable clothes and a pair of running shoes, and take a watch.
- Walking, or running, or using a mixture of both, cover the mile as quickly as you can without getting uncomfortably breathless. It is likely to take between 10 and 20 minutes, so aim for a pace you can keep up. If you have any pain or discomfort, stop. If you are over 55 or have not exercised regularly until recently, and it's the first time you've taken the test, it's best to walk all the way.
- Note down or remember the time it took you to cover the mile and check your results against the figures below.

Minutes taken to cover the mile	Stamina fitness
20 or over	very unfit
15-20	unfit
12-15	fair
10-12	fit
10 or under	very fit

- Repeat the test every month or so to see how you're getting on.

Remember that this test only gives you a rough guide to how fit you are. Your age and lots of other factors will also affect your result. Some younger people may easily cover a mile in under ten minutes. So if you're under 40 and your result is 'very fit' don't give up exercising. To stay fit you need to keep it up. It's not your test result that's important, but the fact that you're feeling fitter as time goes on. If you have to have a break, you'll lose some of the stamina you developed, but you can soon catch up, as long as you remember to start again gradually. You have to keep active, because you can't store fitness.

Eating Well

Food plays a very large part in women's lives. We are the main providers of food – with much of the responsibility for shopping and cooking and for taking care of the health of the family through the food we provide. The food we choose and the way we prepare it is influenced by our budget, and by how much time we have, and if we have a family by their preferences as well as our own. Managing on a tight budget can mean it's hard to eat well – fresh fruit, vegetables and leaner cuts of meat are expensive. Food may be something we cut back on, and women often go without at the expense of other family members or because it doesn't feel worth while to bother for themselves.

The rewards of eating are immediate – it tastes good, it's comforting, it's sociable. There's never been a greater variety of food to choose from, and we are bombarded by messages from the manufacturers making claims about their products and seducing us into buying them. The typical diet in the UK is too rich in fats, especially saturated fats, protein and refined carbohydrates like sugar, cakes, biscuits and confection-ery; and lacking in fibre-rich and starchy foods including fruit, vege-tables, bread, potatoes, pulses and grains. In general, we are overfed but undernourished.

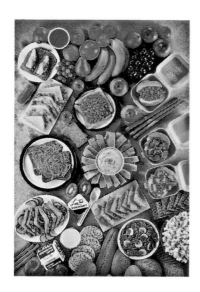

There are clear links between poor diet and a number of health problems – diets too high in fat, especially saturated fat, may lead to heart disease; too much salt has been linked with high blood pressure and strokes in some people; too little fibre may contribute to bowel cancer, constipation and diverticulitis (a common bowel problem); too high an energy intake can lead to obesity; and diabetes, high blood pressure, strokes, heart disease and cancer are all associated with obesity too; and too much sugar may not only contribute to obesity but can cause tooth decay.

Eating habits have been transformed over the last few decades. We're more calorie conscious now than our parents' generation, and many people are beginning to cut down on fat. The last decade has seen a swing from whole milk to skimmed and semi-skimmed milks, and these now make up more than half the milk market; consumption of potatoes has dropped by a third, and we now tend to substitute processed vegetables for fresh; we eat more ready-made meals and take-aways; and while we eat more salads, many of them, like coleslaw, tend to be high on fats and low on vitamins.

Feelings about food

For many women, emotions play a part in shaping their eating patterns. You may use food to make you feel good, to give yourself a treat or reward, because you're bored, to calm your nerves, or as a way of putting off something that needs doing. If you try too hard to please others you may blame yourself for not being good enough, and use food to help relieve the guilty feelings. Sometimes women find themselves blaming their problems on their size and shape – it's easy to believe that everything would be fine if we were slim; or they may try to use their weight as an excuse for not doing things – to avoid the situations that scare them. When women diet excessively to become thin, what they may really be trying to do is disappear. The extremes of these behaviours are a variety of eating disorders (see below).

'When I'm feeling bored or depressed, I find myself standing by the fridge, eating whatever's there. I don't enjoy it, I don't even really taste it – it just gets shovelled in. I can't help myself and I hate myself afterwards.'

'My mum used to ply me with food. Not eating was a way of getting back at her and establishing my own independence.'

You need to try to find other ways to deal with your feelings:

- try not to expect so much of yourself, and put yourself first sometimes
- find some new interests or think about other changes you can make if you're bored
- don't be so hard on yourself and self-critical – focus on your good points and forget or change the rest
- think of other rewards you would enjoy, or choose healthier snacks for your treats.

There are also lots of pressures on us to look and be a certain way. Trying to live up to the images of slim women presented daily through the media can lead us to focus constantly on what we eat, provoking a circle of crash dieting, compulsive eating, weight gain, guilt, and round again. It is easy to believe that all our problems would be solved if only we were slim. We need to find a way to be more accepting of ourselves for who we are, rather than punishing ourselves with obsessive eating regimes.

'If I've eaten too much, I feel guilty and bad about myself. One biscuit and I think that's it, the diet's over. Then I start to binge. It's a vicious circle really.'

Eating disorders

Eating disorders are many and varied and may develop because of the way people feel about themselves. Both men and women are affected, but the problem is far more common among women. Living in a society which prescribes strict guidelines about what is attractive and healthy in terms of size leads many women to feel very pressured about food.

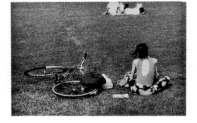

Some eating disorders lead women to feel they are overweight, even though others do not see them as such. They may have been through very traumatic experiences such as sexual abuse or may have been over-controlled as a child, sometimes with great pressure to achieve academically. These sorts of difficulties in childhood may lead to severe forms of eating disorder such as anorexia nervosa or bulimia. Women seem to act out the classic feminine stereotype of extreme self-denial, repression of anger and conflict, desire to remain childlike in body shape, and conformity to the idea of a thin woman. They may feel they have no control over anything except their body.

Anorexia nervosa
- Anorexia nervosa takes the form of severe and deliberate self-starvation and can lead to death. Women with anorexia see their body as much bigger than it actually is.

Bulimia
- Bulimia involves bingeing on different types of food and then purging through either vomiting or taking laxatives. There is a risk of injury to intestines and oesophagus, severe tooth decay from regurgitated stomach acids, and an upset of electrolyte balance. It can damage long-term health or be immediately fatal.

Compulsive eating
- Compulsive eating is yet another eating disorder. A woman may eat to relieve feelings of loneliness, boredom, isolation or frustration, or may use food as a comfort for guilt or depression. Compulsive eating may be to do with insecurity or lack of self-esteem. Most of us have binged at some time to comfort ourselves or cope with our feelings, but, with compulsive eating, food is used in this way on a regular basis, and a lot of weight is gained. For any eating disorder, it's important to get help as soon as possible. The hardest part may be accepting that you have a problem. Your doctor will be able to refer you for counselling or other treatment or support, or see the organisations listed at the end of the book.

Choosing healthy options

Eating well is about enjoying a variety of healthy foods, and choosing to make the changes we want without guilt or pressure. There are lots of suggestions here but you don't have to try them all. Have a go with the ideas that you would find easy and practical, that suit your lifestyle and that you can afford. You don't have to make lots of changes at once – try one or two to start with, and introduce others gradually.

Food provides nutrients to help the body work properly. No single food provides them all in the amounts needed, so it's important to eat a variety of foods. It helps to think of four main food groups, and to choose foods from each of the four groups each day, making sure you don't always select the same ones. Some foods, such as cheese and potatoes, fit into more than one group because of the mixture of nutrients they contain.

Group One

Starchy foods • This group includes foods like bread and rolls, breakfast cereals, chapattis, cornmeal, green bananas, maize, millet, noodles, pasta, potatoes, rice and sweet potatoes.

Group Two

Dairy products • This group includes cheese, fromage frais, milk and yoghurt.

Group Three

Meat, poultry, fish and alternatives • This group includes meat (beef, pork, bacon, lamb), meat products (sausages, beefburgers, meat pies), fish, fish products (fish fingers), poultry (chicken, turkey), beans and lentils (baked beans, chick peas, butter beans, etc.), cheese, eggs, nuts and nut products (like peanut butter), offal (liver, kidney, etc.), texturised vegetable protein (TVP) and other meat alternatives.

Group Four

Vegetables and fruit • This group includes all vegetables such as Brussels sprouts, cabbage, leeks, carrots, okra, parsnips, peppers, potatoes, spinach; salad vegetables

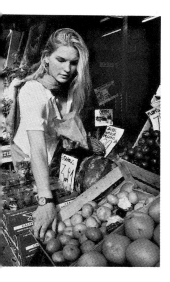

such as cucumber, lettuce, radish, tomato; fruit such as apples, bananas, grapes, mangoes, oranges, soft fruits.

There are a number of simple guidelines to help you enjoy healthy eating:

- enjoy your food
- eat a variety of foods
- eat plenty of foods rich in starch and fibre
- don't eat too much fat
- don't eat sugary foods too often
- look after the vitamins and minerals in your food
- if you drink, keep within sensible limits (see Alcohol, pages 251-261)
- eat the right amount to be a healthy weight

Starch and fibre

It's good to base your meals around the starchy foods in Group 1. They are important because they are filling without providing too many calories, and are a good source of other nutrients. They are usually cheap as well.

In the past, starchy foods have been thought of as fattening, but this is only true if they are served or cooked with fat. For example, a typical helping of boiled potatoes (170 g or 6 oz) provides about 140 calories, while the same weight of chips provides three times as many calories.

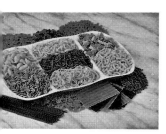

The wholegrain varieties of starchy foods, like wholemeal bread, brown rice, and wholemeal pasta, are a particularly good choice because they are high in fibre, contain more vitamins and minerals, and are more filling. The type of fibre in fruit and vegetables, as well as in oats and beans, may help to reduce the amount of cholesterol in the blood. Because there are different types of fibre, you should include a mixture of fibre-rich foods in your diet. When you have plenty of fibre, you need to make sure you take plenty of fluids too – at least six to eight drinks each day.

Fibre is what some people refer to as roughage. It is only found in foods that come from plants – cereals, grains, seeds, beans, peas, vegetables and fruit. There is no fibre in animal products like meat, cheese or eggs. Bran is a rich source of fibre but it doesn't provide the other nutrients that fibre-rich foods contain. So rather than add bran to food, make sure you eat a good range of the foods mentioned so you get all the fibre you need.

What you need to know about fat

A small amount of fat in the diet is essential for health and to make foods more pleasant to eat. However, we tend to eat far more fat than we need, and this is linked with an increased risk of heart disease (see coronary heart disease, pages 180-181) and can lead to us becoming overweight. Fats have more than twice as many calories, weight for weight, as protein and carbohydrates. There are two types of fats – saturated fats (saturates) and unsaturated fats (unsaturates). The unsaturated group includes polyunsaturated fats and monounsaturated fats. The difference between these types of fat is the chemicals (fatty acids) which they contain.

Saturated fats • These are usually solid at room temperature and are found mainly in animal products from Groups 2 and 3 (dairy products and meat). Some vegetable oils, hard (and some soft) margarines, cooking fats, cakes, biscuits, puddings, savoury snacks and chocolate are also high in saturates. If hydrogenated vegetable fat/oil is included in an ingredients' list, this is a clear indication that the food contains saturates.

Unsaturated fats • These may be liquid at room temperature, and are found in vegetable oils such as sunflower, corn, soya, rapeseed and olive oils, soft margarine labelled 'high in polyunsaturates', nuts and oily fish such as herring, tuna, mackerel, pilchards, sardines and trout.

Cholesterol is found in some foods, but this cholesterol does not have a major effect on the overall amount of blood cholesterol in most people. It is the amount of saturates eaten which is the main influence on blood cholesterol levels, and which may be linked to heart disease.

Our diet tends to contain far too much fat, and too much of the wrong type of fat. The average percentage of food energy derived from fats is currently around 40 per cent, and British Government Health of the Nation targets are seeking to reduce these to no more than 35 per cent in the next ten years, with the proportion coming from saturates reduced to about 11 per cent of food energy. It's fine to include small amounts of unsaturates, but try to cut right down on the saturates. Some fats are easy to spot, like cream, the fat on the outside of meat, butter and margarine, and these are known as visible fats. Other fats are hidden in cakes, chocolate, biscuits, crisps and pastry, so take care with these foods.

Cutting down on fat

There are lots of low-fat versions of the foods in Groups 2 and 3, and these are the ones to go for. The following guidelines may help:

- choose a low or reduced fat spread rather than butter, hard margarine, or ordinary soft margarine. Don't use more because it's lower fat or you'll lose the benefit.
- if you want to carry on using butter, try spreading it more thinly.
- if you use margarine, choose one labelled 'high in polyunsaturates'. These margarines contain the same amount of fat and calories as butter – it's just the type of fat which is different – so, again, spread it more thinly.
- try sometimes not to use any spread, for example, with beans on toast.
- use semi-skimmed or skimmed milk rather than whole milk. Semi-skimmed (half fat) milk tastes like whole (full fat) milk but has had the cream poured off. Skimmed milk has a 'thinner' taste but you soon get used to it. Both have just as much calcium and protein as whole milk but much less fat. Try using skimmed milk in cooking and semi-skimmed in drinks and on cereals. If you use dried milk, read the label and choose a type that hasn't had

vegetable fat added to it. (If you have children under 2, they need to use whole milk.)

- try using low-fat yoghurt or low-fat (labelled less than 1 per cent) fromage frais instead of cream, evaporated milk or condensed milk. If you do use cream, use less and choose single rather than double. Remember that some artificial creams made from vegetable oil have as much fat as dairy cream.

- try half-fat cheese or cottage cheese (natural or flavoured) instead of full-fat hard cheese. Or use smaller portions of stronger-flavoured full-fat hard cheese. Try curd cheese instead of cream cheese.

- make salad dressings with natural yoghurt, herbs, spices, tomato juice, vinegar, or lemon juice rather than mayonnaise or salad cream.

- cut down on crisps, chocolate, cakes, pastries and biscuits.

- eat fish more often. Grill, microwave, steam or bake it rather than deep-frying in batter. Grill fish fingers and fishcakes rather than frying them.

- chicken and turkey are low in fat as long as the skin is removed. Most of the fat is found just under the skin and will easily come away with it.

- buy the leanest cuts of meat you can afford and trim off all the visible fat.

- use smaller quantities of meat and replace it with vegetables, potatoes, or pulses such as beans and lentils.

- try microwaving, steaming, poaching, boiling, or grilling instead of roasting and frying. If you do fry, use a non-stick saucepan and then you may not need to use any fat or oil at all. If you roast, then try 'dry' roasting without added fat, and use a trivet so that all the fat can drain off.

- casseroling and stewing are good ways to cook cheaper cuts of meat. Make sure you remove visible fat, and spoon off any fat that comes to the surface. Remember to take the skin off chicken or turkey before casseroling it. There is no need to fry meat before casseroling, but be aware that it may need a little longer to cook if you do not.

- meat products such as beefburgers and sausages are very fatty. Don't choose them too often, and when you do, buy the ones marked 'low fat' and grill them.

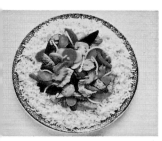

- meat pies, sausage rolls, and other savoury pastry products contain a lot of fat, both in the meat and in the pastry. Don't eat these too often. If you make your own, then use lean meat or low-fat sausagemeat, and make the pastry with a margarine high in polyunsaturates.

- mince is often very fatty even if it doesn't look it. To remove most of the fat, just heat the mince, add cold water, allow to cool slightly, and then you can pour off the fat with the water. The mince can then be cooked in the normal way. Alternatively, use lean mince – in supermarkets, look for the mince labelled 'less than 10 per cent fat'.

- take the fat off the surface of gravy. Let the gravy stand for a few minutes to allow the fat to settle, then spoon it off. Or try using a gravy pourer which is designed to leave fat behind.

- when you use oil and fat for cooking, use as little as possible. Choose one that is high in unsaturates, such as sunflower, soya, corn, rapeseed or olive oil. Measure oil for cooking with tablespoons rather than pouring straight from a container, then gradually try to reduce the number of spoonfuls used.

- try to add as little fat as possible when cooking the spices for meals such as curries. Use an oil that is high in unsaturates instead of fats like ghee, or try half and half. Skim off any fat that comes to the surface.

- when stir-frying, it's best to use a steep-sided, round-bottomed pan like a wok. This allows you to fry your food using only a small amount of oil.

- cut down on chips, but if you do cook them then cut them thick and straight and fry them in oil that is high in unsaturates. Change the oil frequently. Make sure the oil is really hot before frying, drain the chips well once cooked, and blot away any extra oil by using kitchen paper. Or use oven chips instead.

Sugar

Sugar contains only calories and has no other nutrients. You can get all the energy you need from other foods, so you don't need sugar, and too much is the main cause of tooth decay, and may contribute to a general excess energy intake which in turn causes obesity. Read food labels and watch out for sucrose, glucose, dextrose, fructose, and maltose on the ingredients' list of packaged food as they are all forms of sugar, as are honey, syrup, raw sugar, brown sugar, cane sugar, muscovado, and concentrated fruit juice.

Cutting down on sugar

- try drinking tea and coffee without sugar. You might find it easier to cut down a little at a time. If you find that you can't get used to drinks without any sweetness they try using an artificial sweetener.
- when buying soft drinks, try to choose low-calorie ones or unsweetened fruit juices diluted with water or soda water.
- buy fruit tinned in natural juice rather than in syrup.
- try halving the sugar you use in your recipes. It works for most things except jam, meringues and ice-cream.
- beware of sweets, chocolate and cereal bars.
- go easy on biscuits, cakes and all kinds of sweet pastries.
- cut down on jam, marmalade, syrup, treacle and honey.
- avoid buying sugar- and honey-coated breakfast cereals.
- use low-sugar varieties of bought ready-made puddings and desserts.
- dried fruit contains high concentrations of sugar so don't overdo these.

Salt

On average we eat about 13 grams (2.5 teaspoonfuls) of salt a day. About two-thirds of this is added by food manufacturers when the food is processed. Of the remainder, about half is added during cooking or at the table and half is naturally present in food.

We all need some salt, but only about 3 grams (half a teaspoonful) each day. Most of us eat much more salt than we need. Eating too much can lead to high blood pressure. This in turn can cause heart disease (see

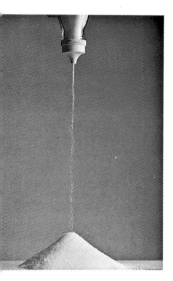

pages 180-181), kidney disease and strokes. So it's worth trying to cut down the amount of salt you eat. At first you might miss the taste of salt, but you'll soon get used to it. Most salt substitutes still contain some salt and will not help you lose the taste for salt. Sea salt contains minute traces of minerals which ordinary salt doesn't, but otherwise there's no difference.

Cutting down on salt

- use less salt in cooking.
- try to get out of the habit of adding salt to food at the table, and always taste food before you do.
- flavour foods with lemon juice, herbs, spices, vinegar or mustard instead of salt.
- cut down on salty snack foods like crisps, salted nuts and other salty nibbles.
- when buying tinned vegetables, choose the ones marked 'no added salt'.
- cut down on salted meats such as bacon, gammon and salt beef.
- stock cubes are very salty. Try making your own stock instead, or use fewer stock cubes and more herbs and spices for flavour.
- watch sauces, especially soya sauce, and foods containing monosodium glutamate.
- use fewer tinned and packet soups. Try making your own homemade soups instead.
- many other ready-prepared savoury dishes can be very salty. Look at the label to find those with less added salt, or try making your own savoury dishes.

The vitamin and mineral maze

Do we need supplements ?

The vitamin market is worth millions and is growing every year. But do we need supplements? Are they really a help or just an expensive hoax? By

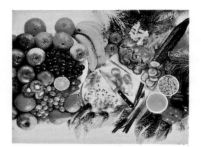

eating a variety of foods from the four food groups (see pages 214-215) you should get all the vitamins and minerals you need. While it's clear that a lack of vitamins and minerals may cause deficiency diseases, too many can also cause problems. To make sure that the foods you eat are as nutritious as possible, foods should be fresh, or stored properly. Keeping fresh foods too long or storing them poorly can lead to a reduction in nutrient content. Fresh food quickly loses its vitamins if it's prepared or cooked in advance – a must for many of us with our busy lives. Convenience foods can be a useful alternative. Frozen, chilled, dried or packaged foods can be as good a source of vitamins and minerals as fresh foods – make sure they are stored properly, and follow any instructions on the pack.

Modern Western lifestyles create problems of their own. Eating habits have been transformed over the last few decades. Today we're calorie conscious and avoid high-fat foods far more than our parents' generation. Cutting down on calories can mean cutting out essential vitamins. For example, in the last decade the level of consumption of whole milk has fallen and, as a consequence, the average intake of Vitamin A has dropped; consumption of potatoes, a rich source of Vitamin C, has also dropped by a third.

As many as a quarter of us are either anaemic or have low iron stores. Women who lose a lot of blood each month with heavy periods are especially at risk, but we all tend to have more periods than our bodies were designed to cope with. Before the days of modern contraception (when women married young and produced babies at regular intervals until their menopause), a woman could expect to have relatively fewer menstrual periods. Women today bleed most months, and their bodies have to work overtime to replace the iron lost with the menstrual blood.

Who benefits from supplements?

While it is not clear if most of us will benefit from supplements, there are certain situations where they are advised. It's best not to take isolated vitamins or minerals without getting advice from your doctor or dietician, because an excess of one can interfere with the absorption of another. It is possible to take so much of some vitamin supplements that they become damaging. If you want to take supplements, multi-vitamin or multi-mineral supplements with a wide and balanced content are probably the best choice, but if you are not sure, do talk to your doctor.

Planning a pregnancy, pregnant or breastfeeding

• Your doctor will advise you about vitamin and mineral supplements, and you shouldn't take them without getting advice. Avoid Vitamin A supplements as too much could harm your baby. Folic acid is special, and you should take folic acid tablets when you're planning a pregnancy, and every day (400 micrograms) until you're 12 weeks pregnant, when you should stop. Even if you're late starting the folic acid, still take it until you're 12 weeks pregnant. Deficiencies in folic acid have been associated with an increased risk of having a child with a neural tube defect such as spina bifida. If you are breast feeding, extra zinc may be helpful.

Eating an inadequate or unbalanced diet

• If you are on a perpetual diet, especially if you're eating fewer than 1,000 calories a day, you risk deficiencies in most vitamins and minerals and should definitely take a good multivitamin/mineral supplement. You may also be short of vitamins and minerals if you exclude large groups of food because of an allergy, because you're a strict vegan, or you just don't like them! As you get older or if you are unwell or convalescing, poor appetite can lead to a restricted diet and supplements can help here too.

If you smoke

• You will probably benefit from a Vitamin C supplement because smoking interferes with your body's absorption of this vitamin. There is some evidence to suggest that Vitamin C is an antioxidant which may slightly reduce a smoker's risk of lung cancer.

If you take regular medication

• Check with your doctor if the medication you take means you need supplements. Certain drugs such as cortisone can lead to deficiencies.

Experts have different views about whether women on the pill have special requirements – it seems that the pill can increase your absorption of Vitamins A and K, but decreases your absorption of Vitamins B6 and B12, folic acid and Vitamin C. However, Vitamin C seems to interfere with the way the body responds to the hormones in the pill and may intensify some of the side-effects. Pill expert Professor John Guillebaud believes that supplements are not necessary but advises those who insist on taking Vitamin C to do so at least four hours before or after your pill. Regular use of over-the-counter medicines such as aspirin may mean you need supplements – check with your doctor or pharmacist.

If you have heavy periods
- You may need extra iron, and Vitamin C will aid its absorption.

If you're vegetarian
- There is evidence that many vegetarian women are short of vitamins. You may miss out on iron, Vitamin B12 and Vitamin D which aids the absorption of calcium.

Labelling and additives

Labelling

By law, most prepared foods must give:

- the name of the food
- a list of ingredients in descending order of weight
- its weight
- how long it can be kept and how to store it
- how to cook or prepare it
- the name and address of the maker, packer or seller
- the place of origin

More food labels now give nutritional information and some make claims

Nutrition information

100g (3½) oz	GIVES YOU
Energy	1475kJ/350 kcal
Protein	11.4g
Carbohydrate	70.3g
(of which sugars)	1.0g
Fat	3.4g
(of which saturates)	0.5g
Sodium	0.2g
Fibre	9.5g

kJ stands for kilojoules – another way of measuring energy.
kcal tells you how many calories there are in 100g of the food.
Carbohydrates include sugar which we should cut down on, and starch, which we could do with more of. In this product the carbohydrates are mostly starch. The **Fat** figure tells you how much fat there is in 100g of the product. Go for products with the lowest amount of saturated fat.
The **Sodium** figure gives you an idea of how much salt is in the food.

that the food has particular benefits. Specific claims like 'low in calories' or 'rich in Vitamin C' have to meet legal conditions. Vaguer claims like 'all natural' are meaningless from a health point of view.

Many manufacturers and food stores are using labels or symbols to identify foods which are 'low fat', 'low sugar' or 'high fibre'. These can be useful as a quick guide but may mean something different on each food and there is no legislation to control their use. For example, a low-fat spread is lower in fat than butter or margarine, but still contains about 40 per cent fat. A low-fat yoghurt, on the other hand, is lower in fat than an ordinary yoghurt and contains less than 1 per cent fat.

A standard format for voluntary nutrition labelling is being introduced in the European Community. In future when a claim such as 'low fat' is made it will be compulsory to give nutrition information on the label. At present it is voluntary. Where available, use the labels to compare similar foods to choose lower-fat, lower-sugar varieties.

Additives

Additives are listed along with the ingredients on most packaged foods. Many additives are shown by their European Community (EC) number (the E number). All of the additives with E numbers have been tested for safety, and passed for use in the EC. Numbers without an E in front are allowed in the UK but may not have been passed for use in all EC countries.

A few people suffer from allergic reactions to some additives, whether natural or synthetic. If this applies to you, the E numbers will help you avoid any additives that cause you problems. Additives are sometimes used when there is no real need for them – for example, food colouring – but most additives have a useful role. Preservatives help to prevent spoilage of food so that it can be stored safely for longer. Consumer pressure to limit additives to essential uses has led to many manufacturers and food chains cutting down on additives.

Are you a healthy weight?

There are enormous pressures on women in our society to look a certain way. Being slim is seen as highly desirable by many people, and around a quarter of us are on a slimming diet at any one time, although the vast majority of us will find that they don't work. Every year we spend £26 billion on slimming products – not including the millions spent on books, tapes and videos. Most popular diet plans fly in the face of a scientific understanding of what fat is, why we gain it and how we can lose it. Metabolism-boosting, chocoholic, Mediterranean, 'spot fat', these are just some of the diets on the market, and the reason they seem so attractive is that they promise a quick and easy way of getting results. Unfortunately, none can provide a fool-proof way of shedding pounds.

If you're trying to lose weight

Check your height and weight against the chart on page 261

- From the chart almost half the adult population in the UK is overweight, and nearly half of these people are fat or very fat. As people get older they tend to put on weight, and, at any age, more women are overweight than men. On the other hand, many women worry about their weight and shape no matter what they weigh, and feel guilty when they eat (see Feelings about food, page 211). Before starting a weight-reduction diet, make sure you really will benefit by losing weight, and be realistic about what weight you should aim for. If you've had any problems with your health, check with your doctor. If you are very fat, or are pregnant or breast-feeding, you may need special help, and your doctor may refer you to a dietician.

Underweight

- Maybe you need to eat a bit more, but go for well-balanced nutritious foods and don't just fill up on fatty and sugary foods. If you are very underweight, see your doctor about it.

OK • Your weight is in the desirable range for health. You're eating the right amount of food, and don't need to restrict your calorie intake. But you need to be sure you're getting a healthy balance in your diet.

Overweight • Your health could suffer so you should try to lose weight.

Fat • It is really important to lose weight for your health.

Very fat • Being this overweight is very serious. You urgently need to lose weight, and you should talk to your doctor, who may refer you to a dietician.

Your weight depends on a number of different factors. If you are trying to lose weight, it's important to take in less energy (calories) from food and do more physical activity. It's easy to underestimate the changes we need to make to shed fat. We're not very good at honestly assessing how much we eat and how active we are, predictably underestimating our food intake and overestimating our activity.

Cutting down on calories

When you eat more energy (calories) than you use up you will put on weight. It's a bit like a balancing act – it is not healthy to be either underweight or overweight. A diet will only work if it reduces your calorie intake. But within that, there are a huge number of healthy foods to choose from – you don't have to live on lettuce leaves and crisp bread! Try to find a new eating pattern that you can live with most of the time, rather than resorting to crash diets or expensive slimming aids – you'll be more successful in controlling your weight in the long run.

Aim to lose 0.5 to 1 kilo (1 to 2 pounds) a week until you reach the 'OK' range. Then maintain this healthy weight by eating a balanced diet, following the guidelines given here, and doing some regular physical activity. Don't weigh yourself too often – there may be fluctuations up and

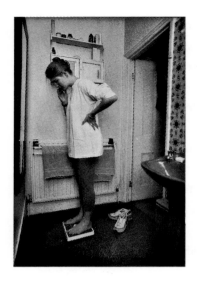

down from day to day thanks to differences in fluid retention, but if you weigh yourself once every two weeks you will be able to detect real changes in your weight.

Try not to be discouraged if your weight loss slows down – everyone is different, and a slow, steady loss is far better for you than a sudden one which you can't maintain.

Short-term weight loss tends to be just that – short term. Permanent weight loss can only be achieved over time. If you feel you need some help to lose weight, ask your friends and family for support and encouragement, or join a slimming group. Like anything else, sharing ideas and problems with other people who are going through the same thing can be a great help.

These general guidelines may help:

- Try to fill up on starchy foods from Group 1, and fruit and vegetables from Group 4 (see pages 216-217) – they have fewer calories and are filling, especially wholegrain foods.
- Cut down on the amount of fat you eat. It has more than twice as many calories as the same weight of starch or protein (see pages 219-221 for ways to cut down on fat).
- Include lower-fat dairy foods (from Group 2) and lean meat and fish (from Group 3) to make sure you don't lose out on minerals, vitamins and proteins when losing weight.
- Cut down on sugary foods such as sweets, chocolate, cakes and biscuits, some of which are also high in fat, and sweetened drinks. Cut out table sugar completely – it contains only calories and no other nutrients, and you can get all the energy you need from other foods (see page 222 for ways to cut down on sugar).
- Avoid sweetened puddings, pastries and pies. You can replace them with fresh fruit or low-fat, low-sugar yoghurt.
- Cut down on alcohol – it contains lots of calories.

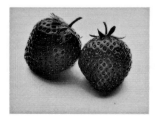

Being active helps

Exercise on its own is not a very effective way of losing weight but, if you combine it with a reduced energy intake through a healthy eating regime, it can work wonders. Regular exercise helps burn up calories, tone slack muscles so your body becomes trimmer, and can help boost your metabolic rate. With exercise, nothing succeeds like success. The more in shape you are, the easier it is to stay that way.

So how does it work?

Appetite control
- Appetite is controlled in the base of the brain and, if you are very inactive, the regulatory system doesn't work properly and your appetite increases. Physical activity raises blood glucose levels, and helps to prevent you feeling hungry, a very good reason for being more active!

Metabolism
- Everyone's metabolism is different, and so too is the way we use up energy and lay down fat. We all know of people who can eat huge amounts of food and are built like stick insects, and others who only have to look at a bar of chocolate to pile on the pounds. Metabolism does play a part in how we use the food we eat. Some people are constantly burning up body fuel – like a car that's always revving – so that the calories they take in are quickly burnt off. Others burn up fewer calories and so need to eat less to replace them.

The amount of energy your body uses when it's resting (just being you) is known as your **basal metabolic rate**. Even when you're asleep or resting, your body is burning calories to sustain itself, though obviously not as much as when you're awake and active. Energy is needed for the chemical changes that turn what you take in (be it air, water or food) into what your body structure needs for life. Air is metabolised into the form of oxygen which can be transported in the bloodstream, and into carbon dioxide which you exhale. Food is metabolised into energy, or fat, or substances needed for the structure of your cells. Toxins and waste products are processed and expelled from your system. It all requires energy.

Your basal metabolic rate is shaped by the following:

the size of your body •

If you have a high ratio of muscle to fat, you'll burn up calories faster than if you have a small muscle mass. This is because the cells in muscle tissue are metabolically active whereas fat cells are not, so the more muscle tissue you have, the more energy you use. This seems to be the case even when you're not being active, because resting muscles also need energy to maintain themselves. That's why men have a higher metabolic rate than women and use more energy – they usually have more muscle to sustain.

your age •

Your basal metabolic rate decreases with age. New muscle and bone tissue are constantly being made but, as you get older, you need less energy because you lose muscle mass and your body functions slow down.

your hormones •

The action of certain glands, in particular the thyroid and adrenal glands, can slow down or speed up your metabolic rate. If the thyroid is over- or under-active it can upset your basal metabolic rate, causing you to gain or lose weight rapidly.

While there is little you can do to change these factors, there is one way to boost your metabolism – be more physically active. Recent research shows that exercise can speed up your metabolic rate by increasing the pace at which you burn calories, and it also peps up your basal metabolic rate by transforming your body structure.

How does exercise help?

By building muscle, exercise makes your energy metabolism more effective. Muscle burns up calories simply to maintain itself, so the more muscle tissue you build up, the higher your basal metabolic rate will be, even when you're not exercising!

Energy transforms your muscle cells so that they metabolise energy in a different way by increasing the number of energy processors known as mitochondria. Energy is created in the mitochondria through a chemical reaction that begins when your body converts the carbohydrate and fat from food into a sort of chemical fuel called adenosine triphosphate (ATP). ATP then serves as the power source for muscular movement.

For reasons which physiologists do not quite understand, the bigger and more numerous your mitochondria become, the more you tend to burn fat instead of carbohydrate to supply your muscles with energy, which is great news for anyone trying to shift excess pounds. It also means that your metabolism becomes more effective during exercise. If you rely on your carbohydrate store to provide energy you can't keep going very long. A nine-stone woman stores only about 1,800 calories' worth of energy in carbohydrates – enough to last for just about two hours of heavy exercise, and then she's done for. But the same woman has enough fat on her body to provide an inexhaustible supply of energy. It seems that regular aerobic exercise may increase levels of a muscle compound called myoglobin, which helps speed the transfer of oxygen from the blood to muscle fibres. The increase in blood flow and enzyme activity improves the ability of muscles to break down fats and carbohydrates – especially fats – which helps you to lose weight. This is why if you're out of shape, your body relies more on carbohydrate fuel so you run out of steam more quickly, but if you're in shape you can process your fat.

So, if you've been trying to lose weight through exercise for a while you reach a point where everything seems to speed up. It feels as though you've boosted your metabolism and in a way you have – you've changed the way you metabolise energy.

How much energy do you use?

Calories per hour		Activity
80-100	•	Sedentary activities e.g. reading, writing, sitting, watching TV.
110-160	•	Light activities e.g. washing up, ironing, walking slowly, office work involving some activity like filing.
170-240	•	Moderate activities e.g. making beds, sweeping, light gardening, walking moderately fast.
250-350	•	Vigorous activities e.g. walking fast, bowling, riding, heavy gardening, carrying small children.
350+	•	Strenuous activities e.g. swimming, running or cycling quickly, playing squash.

Different shapes and sizes

Fat is a vital part of your body and performs different functions in different places – on the soles of your feet, a dense layer of fat acts as padding; behind your eyeballs, fatty deposits aid the function of the nerves in your eyes; and you couldn't survive without the fat dispersed around your brain. Individuals not only lay down fat at different speeds, but store it in different places – fat deposits form both under the skin, known as subcutaneous fat – and between the organs in the abdomen – intra-abdominal fat, leading to two different shapes – the round 'apple' and the bottom-heavy 'pear'.

You can calculate whether you're an apple or a pear by comparing your hip size to your waist. If your waist measurement is more than 75 per cent of your hips, then you're an apple and have a relatively high level of intra-abdominal fat, known as 'central fat distribution'. Pear shapes carry subcutaneous fat in what physiologists call a 'peripheral fat distribution'.

Central fat distribution carries more of a risk to your health, making you more predisposed to coronary heart disease, strokes, diabetes, gallstones, and possibly breast cancer. Some research shows that you are more likely to suffer from fertility problems. 'Peripheral' fat carries less risk, but also seems to be less responsive to dieting.

Men tend to store their fat intra-abdominally, while women store more of it under our skin. When men do store fat subcutaneously, it's more likely to settle on their stomach or back, while we usually carry it on our hips and thighs – although pregnant women tend to lay down fat stores on their arms and shoulders. For reasons as yet undiscovered, you're more likely to have a central fat distribution if you smoke or drink a lot of alcohol than if you don't.

The way that female fat is distributed predisposes us to cellulite. 80 per cent of women complain about dimpled fat deposits on bums, thighs and tums, including those who are not overweight! Cosmetic counters are full of massages and rubs that claim to break it down. There are as many explanations of cellulite as there are products to get rid of it. However, most physiologists dispute the claim that cellulite is any different from normal fat. The characteristic dimpled appearance of cellulite is more to do with the structure of women's skin than the texture of the fat itself. The dimples are caused by the connective fibres which run from the skin to muscles and, when fat deposits lie underneath the skin, they act like buttons on a cushion producing a dimpled surface. Men don't get this so much because they lay down less fat on their thighs, have differently arranged connective tissue and have stronger and thicker skin that is less likely to dimple. The creams that you can buy at extortionate prices certainly can't dissolve away the fat, and in so far as they work at all it's because they tone and tighten the skin.

Your body shape and metabolism is partly down to your genes. Obesity sometimes seems to run in families, which some scientists believe may be due to a 'thrifty' gene which allows them to burn up only a small proportion of the energy expended by the rest of us. But a lot of family similarities in size are more likely to be owing to the eating habits which we learn at home. Although genes might predispose you to a particular body shape or weight, it's still your lifestyle and eating patterns that have the greater influence.

Smoking

Who smokes?

The number of people smoking in Britain has fallen quite dramatically over the last twenty years. Today, around a third of men and women smoke, compared with more than 46 per cent in 1972. The gap in rates of smoking which used to exist between men and women has gradually closed. Nearly half of Britain's 14 million smokers are now women. This is because more young girls than boys start smoking, while at the same time more men than women quit. Men are twice as successful at stopping, and women who do give up are more likely to go back to smoking. Women have caught up with men not just in the number of us who smoke, but in how many cigarettes we smoke.

In the UK, the highest rates of smoking are among the poorest section of the population. Almost twice as many working-class women as professional women smoke. The teenage girls who take up smoking tend to have a low self-esteem, are more likely to be underachievers at school, and have a background of social disadvantage. Women most likely to smoke are those with low incomes, low-status jobs or who are unemployed, especially single parents with dependent children – the ones in fact who can least afford to. These facts are true across the world.

Why do women smoke?

Taking up smoking

Many of the young girls starting to smoke see it as desirable and generally socially acceptable. They may use it as a way of rebelling, or in an attempt to appear grown up. It may help them feel attractive and sexually mature, making it easier for them to develop relationships with boys. Peer-group pressure also plays a big part at this age, and if parents and other adults around them smoke this also influences them to smoke.

Keeping the lid on feelings

A few years on, the women who smoke are often the ones caring for young children, possibly single-handed for much if not all of the time, and having to manage with little money. They use cigarettes to cope when they feel low, tired, on edge and isolated.

'Smoking gives me a break – a legitimate reason to sit down for five minutes with a cup of tea without someone wanting something or interrupting.'

'When the kids get me down, I light up a cigarette to calm me down. It's better than shouting at them. They usually give me a bit of peace for five minutes.'

'I call in on my neighbour and we have a coffee and a cigarette together. It gives us an excuse for a natter, and breaks the monotony of the day.'

It seems that we smoke as a way of coping. It helps us get through the day and gives some short-lived relief from the stress of work or family, or more often both. Women often describe smoking as their one and only luxury – the one thing they buy for themselves when money is tight, and the thing they'd find it hardest to do without. Women much more than men believe that they actually need to smoke. The tranquillising or relaxing effects of smoking may help us to dampen down feelings of anger or frustration which might otherwise lead to unacceptable or undesirable behaviour, anxiety and possibly depression. In order to avoid shouting at the boss, retaliating with our partner or getting mad with the children, we light up a cigarette. In a way, women chose it as the lesser evil – a way of smoothing things over and making sure everyone else is all right despite the enormous personal costs in terms of their own health.

What's the damage?

Smoking is still the largest single cause of preventable and premature death in this country. Quitting is the single most effective step you can take to improve your health. Illness related to smoking was estimated to cost the NHS over £500 million in 1988, and to this must be added the huge cost to society from the loss of many working days.

Heart attacks, lung cancer and chronic bronchitis are the big three diseases caused by cigarette smoking. But smoking has also been linked to many other conditions, including cancer of the mouth, larynx, oesophagus, pancreas, bladder and cervix, reduced fertility, low birth weight babies, and a greater chance of babies dying around the time of birth. Smoking can also lead to early menopause, which in turn is linked with osteoporosis and bone fracture.

At least 150,000 people in the UK die because of smoking each year: 90 per cent of deaths from lung cancer and bronchitis, and around a quarter of all deaths from coronary heart disease are caused by smoking. Worldwide, smoking was estimated to cause 300,000 deaths among women in 1985 – 41 per cent from cardiovascular disease, 41 per cent from lung cancer, and 18 per cent from chronic lung disease. The Imperial Cancer Research Fund (ICRF) finds there are 150,000 deaths annually in the UK from smoking: 400 a day, one every four minutes.[1]

[1] **The Lancet,** 22 May 1992.

| Lung cancer | • | Women are starting to smoke at a younger age, a larger number of women smoke more than twenty cigarettes a day, and there has been an increase in the total number of cigarettes smoked, leading to a greater lifetime exposure to tobacco. Smoking up to fourteen cigarettes a day means you have eight times the risk of dying from lung cancer. ICRF figures show that 12,345 women died from lung cancer in 1990. Lung cancer is almost always fatal – fewer than one person in ten diagnosed with lung cancer survives for longer than five years. |

| Chronic bronchitis and emphysema | • | These two conditions commonly occur together. They are a major cause of ill health, leading to increasing and gradually debilitating breathlessness and severe chest infections. About seven out of ten cases of chronic bronchitis and emphysema among women are caused by smoking. Fortunately, these diseases are on the decline because fewer people smoke today, air is less polluted and there are better treatments available. |

| Cervical cancer | • | The earlier you start smoking and the more you smoke, the greater your chance of developing cervical cancer. If your partner smokes, this also increases your risk slightly. Nicotine has been found in the cervical secretions of smokers, and there appears to be a link between smoking and all stages of pre-cancer to fully developed cervical cancer. Around one-third of all cases of cervical cancer are linked to smoking. |

| Other cancers | • | Among women, about half of all cancers of the mouth, larynx and oesophagus, and a third of all cancers of the pancreas and bladder are related to smoking. |

| Cardiovascular disease | • | Smoking is a major cause of coronary heart disease. A woman who smokes twenty cigarettes a day is at least twice as likely to die from a heart attack as a non-smoker, irrespective of any other risk factors. For women on the pill, smoking is an added risk – a woman who smokes and takes oral contraceptives has ten times the risk of a heart attack, stroke or other cardiovascular disease than a woman who neither smokes nor takes the |

pill. If you stop smoking, you greatly reduce your risk of heart attack and stroke within a few years.

When you're pregnant

Women smokers have more difficulty becoming pregnant, and once they are pregnant, smoking is definitely harmful. Most women know that there are risks both to themselves and to their baby if they smoke during pregnancy. Lots of women use pregnancy as a time to give up smoking, around 30 per cent of women smokers spontaneously quitting when they first find out they are pregnant. But while most women are anxious that pregnancy and birth will be trouble free, and that their baby will be healthy, some of them find it hard to give up smoking. Being made to feel guilty about it will probably not help them to quit. What's needed most is lots of support and encouragement to help them give up and stay off cigarettes, for their own health as well as the baby's.

Smoking during pregnancy can affect the development of the baby, cause it to grow more slowly, and lead to low birth weight and a greater risk that the baby will die around the time of birth. Smoking has an adverse effect on the placenta which may reduce the oxygen supply and the nutrition to the developing foetus. Women who smoke fifteen or more cigarettes a day during pregnancy have at least twice the risk of miscarriage, twice as many low birth weight babies, leading to significantly more stillbirths, and one-third greater chance of their baby dying during the first month of life. Even smoking a few cigarettes is harmful.

The earlier you give up smoking the better, ideally, when you are thinking about getting pregnant. Giving up smoking during the first sixteen weeks of pregnancy will be a particular help in protecting your baby from slow growth and low birth weight, but it's never too late. Your baby will benefit from you giving up smoking even as late as the thirtieth week of gestation. Once your baby is born, a smoky environment can increase the risk of cot death and chest infections, especially in the first year, so it's much better if you and your partner don't smoke.

If you take the oral contraceptive pill

If you smoke and take the pill you have a greatly increased risk of cardiovascular disease such as heart disease or stroke (see cardiovascular disease, page 180). This gives you every incentive to give up smoking, but if not, you may want to consider some other form of contraception (see pages 68-73).

Giving Up Smoking

You can do it!

The good news is that many people do succeed in giving up. There are around 10 million ex-smokers in the UK today. You may be one of the lucky people who decide to quit and just do it. Around 90 per cent of people giving up smoking do so without any help. The most important thing is to make the decision to give up and believe that you will benefit from doing so. You need to feel confident that you will be able to stop, and support from others can be a big help here. Planning to give up and thinking through how and when you will do so will mean you are more likely to succeed.

Finding the motivation

Wanting and believing

It probably sounds rather obvious, but being really motivated to give up smoking will go a long way towards helping you succeed. Wanting to give up and believing that you can do it are two of the ways to success. Unfortunately, women are more likely than men to believe they actually need to smoke and to lack confidence in their ability to quit. Many see smoking as a much needed comfort or a crutch to help them cope with the pressures or frustrations in their life, to help them control negative feelings, give them the strength to be successful in their careers, or to provide the necessary willpower to stay thin. Believing any or all of these may be enough to keep women smoking.

For some of us, knowing that our smoking is harming others, especially our children, may be enough motivation to give up. But being made to feel guilty about smoking, without any encouragement or support, may just leave us feeling helpless and bad about ourselves for not having more willpower. Pressure from family to give up smoking may actually make it harder rather than easier to succeed. It's not enough to stop smoking just to please someone else – we need to want it for ourselves.

Counting the benefits

However much you feel you need cigarettes, the truth is that giving up is the single most important thing you can do for your health. You will quickly begin to feel better and have fewer problems like breathlessness and coughing.

'I was very surprised to find I felt so much better so quickly. I'd just accepted my cough as a fact of life – within weeks it was gone.'

And the longer you don't smoke, the more you will benefit. After only one year without smoking, the extra risk of heart disease is reduced by half; and after fifteen years your chance of dying prematurely is almost the same as for someone who has never smoked. If you're in your 30s when you give up, you can expect to gain around three extra years of life. It's never too late – even giving up in your 60s will increase your life expectancy by a year. And it's not just heavy smokers who will benefit from giving up smoking. Even if you don't smoke much or you don't smoke regularly, you will still be more healthy (and, incidentally, less likely to become a heavy smoker) if you give up.

Besides being such a positive thing to do for your own health, giving up smoking will help to protect the health of your family, friends, and anyone else who comes into contact with you and your smoking. And of course there will be other benefits too, like saving money. You know it makes sense to give up, so how can you find the motivation you need? Don't try to convince yourself that you are not at risk, or that the damage has already been done. Think through how you personally will benefit, both now and in the future, if you stop smoking:

- your health will improve immediately, and for every year you don't smoke, you will reduce your chance of becoming ill through smoking.
- you will protect the health of the people around you, and will set a good example to your own and other people's children.
- giving up smoking before you get pregnant or in the first three months will reduce your risk of having a low birth weight baby. Quitting at any time during pregnancy will benefit you and your baby.
- you'll save money. At current prices, if you've been smoking twenty cigarettes a day, giving up will save you around £17.50 a week, or £900 a year.
- your clothes, hair and breath will smell fresher, and, providing other people around you don't smoke, your home, car, and office will be cleaner and sweeter smelling too.
- you will feel more in control of your life, and should get a sense of achievement from succeeding in giving up.

Fear of gaining weight

It's a fact of life that most women want to be thin. Society values us for what we look like rather than who we are. Pressures from the fashion industry and the media tell us that thin is sexy and beautiful and advertisements are designed to persuade us that smoking will make us thin and keep us that way.

'My thinness gives me self-respect – a feeling that I am in control.'

Women much more than men see smoking as a way to lose weight, and worry about gaining weight if they quit. Nicotine tends to suppress the appetite, and it's tempting to replace cigarettes with food, especially at first. The average weight gain for women is 8 pounds. Yet not everyone puts on weight when they stop smoking. In fact only about one person in three who gives up smoking will gain any weight, while others will stay the same or may even lose weight. If you do gain a few pounds at first, with sensible eating you will be able to lose it again if you wish. A few extra pounds in weight will not do anything like the same harm as continuing to smoke.

Worries about gaining weight can be a big factor in preventing women from giving up smoking. Yet again, cigarettes are viewed as a price worth paying, a benefit here and now as opposed to some unknown problem in the future. If worrying about your weight is stopping you from giving up smoking, talk to your doctor about how you can be extra careful to avoid putting on weight, or share ideas with friends who have managed to quit successfully. It really is worth doing.

Thinking about your smoking

It's helpful to spend a bit of time thinking about your own smoking behaviour – what are your main reasons for smoking? When do you smoke? What are your main worries about giving up? This will give you a better chance of planning different ways to cope when you quit.

If you have been smoking for any length of time, you may well have become dependent on nicotine. It is a highly addictive drug, and withdrawal symptoms can be unpleasant. When you smoke a cigarette, blood levels of nicotine rise, and then fall soon after giving you a feeling of withdrawal. By smoking, you avoid the feeling of discomfort caused by withdrawal, giving the illusion that smoking has made you feel good.

As well as the part that addiction plays, smoking rapidly becomes a habit. You may associate smoking with certain everyday activities such as drinking tea, coffee or alcohol, taking a break, or chatting to a friend on the 'phone. These habits build up over time, and may take a while to break with when you quit. Being aware of the 'danger' times when you are most likely to want a cigarette will help you to avoid such situations altogether or to stiffen your resolve against smoking at these times. Gradually, you will find that the desire to smoke weakens as you get used to new habits and ways of dealing with situations.

Planning to quit

It's best not to give up smoking on impulse, without any preparation. You will have more chance of success if you think about it carefully and make some plans. If you've tried giving up before, think about what the pitfalls were so you can try to find ways round them this time. It may help to keep a diary for a few days to help pinpoint the times when you smoke, your reasons for having a cigarette at different times of the day, and the moods that are associated with your smoking. Once you've filled in the diary for a few days, you may be able to see patterns to your smoking that will help you work out some strategies for giving up.

Coping strategies

Have a few ideas to cope with the tough times while you are giving up. It may be helpful to avoid your smoking friends just now, and seek out those who don't smoke and who will encourage and support you in your efforts to quit. Try to keep busy without over-stretching yourself – if you find you need something to do with your hands, take up doodling or knitting. Switching to soft drinks may help if you associate coffee, tea or alcohol with smoking. And although it's not a good idea to use food as a substitute for cigarettes, it may help to have some healthy snacks and nibbles like raw carrots, celery and fruit at hand. Anything that will provide you with delaying tactics or something to do till the craving goes away is worth a try. Make life as easy as you can for yourself, and ask your family and friends to be understanding if you're irritable or feeling down. Most important, plan some rewards to give yourself as you succeed in giving up.

Choosing a day

It's never the perfect time, but some days may be easier than others. Try to avoid a time when you know you'll be under a lot of pressure, seeing friends who smoke, bored with nothing to occupy you, or in a situation which you particularly associate with smoking, such as a dinner-party or the pub. Instead, choose a time which will give you every chance of success – for example, when you've plenty to keep you busy but not a great deal of stress, or when you're going to be with non-smoking friends or in a situation where smoking is not allowed. Set a date in the next two weeks, so that you strike while your motivation is high. Decide to give up, choose a day, and go for it.

Finding support

Some people find giving up smoking is easier than they expected. If so, that's great – go ahead and enjoy your success and sense of achievement. You deserve it! If it proves harder, you may want to get some kind of help or support to get you through the worst stages.

Family and friends •

What you need are people around you who will not only encourage you to give up, but will support your efforts to do so. Ask them to help you succeed by making sure they don't smoke when you're around, they don't offer you cigarettes and they share in your celebrations when you manage to quit. Giving up with someone else, perhaps your partner or a friend, may be especially helpful. You can support each other through the bad times, and encourage each other to keep going.

Groups • Although most people give up on their own, some smokers, especially women, find it helpful to go to a stop-smoking group of some kind. These may be provided at your GP surgery (see GP services, pages 303-305) or through some other health, local authority or voluntary service. You can find out about smoking groups in your area through you – community health council, health promotion service, or Citizens' Advice Bureau (and see the addresses at the end of the book).

A group will offer you the chance to find out more about smoking and ways you can try to give up. You will be able to share ideas with people who are going through the same thing, and support each other.

Telephone quitlines • These may be useful if you need to talk to someone about your efforts to give up smoking. 'Quit' offers a nationwide telephone helpline for smokers who wish to quit and for ex-smokers who want extra support. You will speak to one of their trained counsellors who will offer supportive and non-judgmental advice. They can also send you free information about giving up smoking, and can refer you to a stop-smoking group or one-to-one counsellor near you.

No Smoking Day Campaign

No Smoking Day (NSD) is held in March each year and is organised by several health promotion agencies and charities. It provides a focus for lots of local activity to do with encouraging smokers to quit and helping them do so. Since 1984 it has helped 400,000 smokers to give up. If you think getting involved in some activities linked to NSD will be useful for you, get in touch with your local health promotion service (in the phone book) to find out what's going on in your area.

Aids and therapies

Your own determination will be the best aid you have to giving up smoking. But the following aids and therapies may be some help if you haven't managed to quit on your own. Remember, though, that many of them are expensive, and there is no guarantee they will work:

Patches • Patches are placed on your skin and contain nicotine in a reservoir which seeps through into your body at a constant rate. You gradually decrease the dosage you are receiving. The price is around £130 for three months, from pharmacists.

Nicorette • Nicorette is chewing-gum containing nicotine which helps to reduce withdrawal symptoms. Some people find it hard to stop using the gum. Price around £5.50 a box of 30 pieces.

Tabmint • Tabmint is chewing-gum which leaves an unpleasant taste in your mouth if you smoke. Price around £2.75 for 12 pieces, from pharmacists.

Hypnotherapy • Hypnotherapy. A qualified hypnotist may be able to help you give up smoking, but you may need several sessions which can make it expensive (see Alternative therapies, page 29). Price around £25 a session.

Acupuncture • Acupuncture treatment involves needles, or a small stud applied to the ear which may ease craving when pressure is applied (see Alternative therapies, pages 315-316).

Stopping and staying stopped

Although some people find giving up very easy, many people do find the withdrawal from tobacco unpleasant. There will be times when you feel tempted to have a cigarette. Don't make the mistake of believing that just one won't hurt. You will probably find it very hard to smoke on an occasional basis, especially if you've been used to smoking more. Try to resist the desire for a cigarette, relax or find something else to do instead. If you do weaken and have one, don't let that be an excuse to start again. Instead, think about what you could have done to avoid it, keep up your determination, and think about where you can find extra support. Remember that it may take a great deal of time to learn to do without cigarettes.

Try to take each day at a time, and enjoy a feeling of achievement with every day that goes by without your smoking. During the first days and weeks, you may experience all sorts of different feelings and symptoms. If you are worried by any of them, or they persist, see your doctor. Remember that these symptoms and feelings are a part of the process of giving up for many people, and they should only last a short while, so try not to let them discourage you. Instead, think back over your coping strategies, and put them into action.

Withdrawal symptoms

- These may be uncomfortable, but the most severe should only last five to ten days, and things should get easier within three to four weeks.

Craving

- Most smokers will experience some craving at first, but the feelings will go in time if you don't smoke. If you find it very hard to bear, you may want to consider using one of the aids described above.

Cough

- This may be more noticeable than when you were smoking, because the cilia, the small hairs which remove debris from the respiratory system, become more active, sometimes causing a temporary cough.

Sleep problems

- If you find it hard to sleep, try some relaxation exercises (see page 31), and be as active as you can to tire yourself out.

Tiredness

- If you're tired, take every opportunity to rest or sleep, and go easy on yourself.

Feeling low • Remember that giving up smoking may take a lot of energy and may leave you feeling low for a time. Talking through how you feel with a friend, or someone who has given up and knows how it feels may help.

If you don't succeed first time

Around 70 per cent of smokers make one or two attempts to give up smoking before succeeding. Others try even more times – nearly one in ten will quit six or more times before they manage to give up for good. Every time you try to give up, you are actually more likely to succeed in the end. So don't feel too disheartened if you don't manage it first time. Give yourself time to think about what went wrong and build up your motivation before trying again.

Other people's smoke

Only 15 per cent of the smoke from a cigarette is inhaled by the smoker, the rest goes into the surrounding air and other people can breathe it in. Because that air contains tobacco smoke it can be bad for your health. The danger to your health from other people's cigarette smoke is greatest if you are confined in an enclosed space with smokers for much of your time – particularly if you live or work with someone who smokes. Being in a smoky environment can cause all sorts of discomfort and irritation – your throat may feel dry or sore, your nose becomes blocked-up, and your eyes may water (especially if you wear contact lenses); you may become wheezy, dizzy or develop a headache. Worse still, several hundred non-smokers die each year from lung cancer caused by passive smoking, and there may also be a link with heart disease.

If you are pregnant, your baby will be at risk if you are exposed to passive smoking, even if you don't smoke yourself. You should try to avoid smoky places, and ask your family and friends to avoid smoking when you're there. If your partner smokes, this would be a good opportunity to encourage him or her to quit.

When babies and small children are exposed to cigarette smoke in their own homes, they are more likely to suffer from particular health problems than those in smoke-free homes. Babies are more prone to asthma, bronchitis and middle-ear infections and are admitted to hospital with respiratory infections such as pneumonia more often. Older children may get more sore throats, coughs, wheezing and are more likely to have respiratory problems than children from non-smoking families.

There has been a definite change in public opinion in recent years. Non-smokers are asserting their right not to have to live or work in smoky conditions, by ensuring that all enclosed public places are smoke-free. In the UK, it is mainly left to employers and those controlling public buildings and transport services to decide whether or not smoking should be restricted. Many public places, including schools, hospitals, restaurants, buses, cinemas and pubs have now introduced smoking policies, either banning smoking altogether or restricting it to certain areas, and these have proved popular with smokers and non-smokers alike. Many workplaces have also introduced no-smoking policies (see Health care at work, pages 325-326).

Alcohol

Choosing to drink

Most women drink sensibly, and more women than men, around one in seven, choose not to drink at all. Nearly half of all women in the UK have a drink at least once a week. Men are much more likely to be heavy drinkers and women much more likely to be occasional drinkers. A study by the HEA in 1992 found that 6 per cent of women questioned had recently exceeded the recommended limit, compared with more than 20 per cent of men.

Women drink alcohol for all sorts of reasons. Many of us use alcohol in a positive way, when relaxing with friends, going out socially, with meals, or just to unwind at the end of a busy day. Sometimes there are pressures on us to drink more than we want – it may be seen as unsociable to refuse a drink or opt for something non-alcoholic.

For a variety of reasons, lesbian women may drink more alcohol than heterosexual women – they may be subjected to more stress and pressure because of their sexuality. The places where lesbians tend to meet each other and socialise are often alcohol-centred venues such as clubs, pubs and parties, which also encourages drinking. It may be more difficult for a lesbian to find a safe and supportive environment to seek help for a drink problem, although self-help groups do exist in larger cities.

There seems to be an increase in drinking amongst women, probably partly because women's disposable income has risen, the real price of alcohol has fallen, and alcohol is more easily available in corner shops, supermarkets and off-licences. Also, women have been targeted by the alcohol industry's marketing and advertising campaigns which portray women who drink as glamorous, successful, sexy and liberated.

What happens when you drink?

When you have a drink, the alcohol is absorbed from the stomach and intestines into the bloodstream, and circulates round the body. If you have recently eaten, or eat and drink together, the alcohol is absorbed more slowly, and is less likely to irritate the stomach lining. It is in the liver that most alcohol is broken down into energy and other products. It can process about 1 unit of alcohol in an hour, and any more than that will remain in your bloodstream, affecting your feelings, judgement and self-control.

Mood changes • Alcohol may sometimes make you feel relaxed and happy, but it can also make you feel low, tired and argumentative. Alcohol is actually a depressant, not a stimulant, and many women who drink heavily may suffer from anxiety and depression. Drinking itself may cause these feelings, or you may be drinking because of them.

Hangovers • The more you drink, the more likely you are to get a hangover – common symptoms are thirst, nausea and headache. The most common cause of a hangover is dehydration, because alcohol makes us pass lots of water. Drinking plenty of water can help prevent one. Certain drinks are more likely to cause a hangover – congeners are chemicals which are mixed with some drinks to give them colour and taste, and can cause hangovers. Red wine and whisky, for example, contain more congeners than white wine or vodka.

With other drugs • Alcohol and medicines do not mix, so check with your doctor. The oral contraceptive pill may slow down the rate at which you absorb alcohol, so you may find the effects of drinking alcohol last longer. If you are taking drugs such as sleeping pills, tranquillisers, anti-depressants or anti-histamines, alcohol can be particularly dangerous. It may also interfere with the action of other drugs, reducing their effectiveness.

Your menstrual cycle • You may find you become intoxicated more quickly than usual just before your period and during ovulation.

How much is sensible?

Most experts agree that a little alcohol may do you good, both physically and mentally, and certainly won't harm you. There is some evidence that women who drink fewer than 13 units a week may actually have fewer heart attacks and live longer than women who don't drink at all. How much you can drink safely depends on many individual characteristics to do with your body weight and size, whether you have eaten, how generally fit you are, and drinking behaviour such as how quickly and

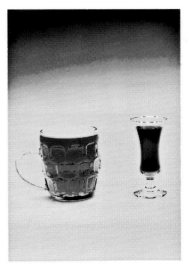

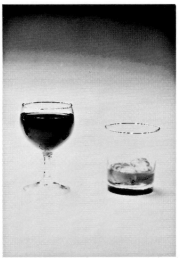

how often you drink. What is clear is that, above a sensible limit, the more you drink the greater the risk of accidents and damage to your health.

So what is a sensible limit for you? There are clear differences in the amounts that men and women can drink safely. Women are generally smaller than men, and have more fat and less water in their bodies. Since alcohol is distributed in body fluid, the alcohol a woman drinks will be more concentrated in her system. This means that women tend to get drunk faster and feel the effects for longer. Women also have smaller livers, and so are more likely to risk damage at lower levels of drinking. You may find that alcohol affects you more if you are smaller or younger or less used to drinking. As you get older, too, the water content of your body declines so fewer drinks may make your alcohol content more concentrated.

The medically recommended sensible guideline for women is not more than 14 units spread throughout the week, with one or two drink-free days. (For men, the limit is 21 units a week.) If you are pregnant, the advice is to drink less than this or give up alcohol altogether.

So how many units do different drinks contain? Well, it depends on their strength and the measure you consume. The following provides a rough guideline.

These drinks (in pub measures) each contain roughly one unit of alcohol. Some drinks contain more than one unit, for example:

$\frac{1}{2}$ pint strong beer, lager, cider (6 per cent ABV) = 2 units
$\frac{1}{2}$ pint extra strong beer, lager, cider (9 per cent ABV) = 2 $\frac{1}{2}$ units
A cocktail (with 3 or 4 measures of alcohol) = 3 or 4 units
A bottle of wine (75 cl) at 11 per cent ABV = about 8 units

(ABV stands for 'Alcohol by volume' and appears on most labels).

Home measures are likely to be much more generous than pub measures, so look carefully at how much you have in your glass and work out how many units it may contain. Home-made beers and wines may be stronger than commercial products. Abroad, the measures may also be larger.

What's the harm?

Fewer than 14 units a week spread throughout the week

Your risk of cancer from drinking:

Low

15 – 34 units a week

Your risk of cancer from drinking:

Increased, particularly if you are a smoker

35 or more units a week

Your risk of cancer from drinking:

Very high, particularly, if you are a smoker

Drinking can be sociable and enjoyable, but too much alcohol can lead to health problems. Experts don't know for sure which diseases are actually caused by alcohol and which are related more loosely, but it is clear that drinking over the sensible limit increases you chances of getting ill. If you are drinking too much you are more likely to suffer from gastritis, ulcers, pancreatitis, blood disorders and malnutrition. The more you drink, the more you risk developing problems. The following conditions are all related to excess alcohol.

Cancer

Heavy drinking (35+ units a week) is associated with an increased incidence of cancer of the mouth and throat (especially if you smoke as well), the liver, colon and rectum. The more you drink, the greater the risk. There is also some evidence that alcohol slightly increases your risk of breast cancer.

Cardiovascular disease

Heart disease •

There is some evidence that light or moderate drinking (fewer than 13 units for women) may mean you are less likely to suffer a heart attack, possibly partly owing to its association with increased concentrations of high density lipoprotein cholesterol which protects against coronary heart disease. But excess drinking can lead to high blood pressure, which increases you chance of heart disease. And heavy drinking over a number of years can lead to weakening of the heart muscle, a condition called cardiomyopathy, which may result in heart failure.

Blood pressure and • Drinking over a number of years contributes to high blood pressure.
strokes Alcohol consumption over the recommended levels may be associated
with two to four times the risk of death from stroke through raising blood
pressure.

Liver damage

Liver damage is common in people who drink excessive amounts of
alcohol. In most heavy drinkers, liver cells will die and be replaced with
fatty tissue. As many as a third may go on to develop fibrous liver tissue, a
severe condition known as cirrhosis. This is irreversible and stops the liver
from functioning normally. You are ten times more likely to die from
cirrhosis if you drink heavily compared with not drinking at all. In 1991,
around 1,350 women died from cirrhosis of the liver, and death rates
from this have been increasing over the last twenty years.

Brain function

Alcohol can slow down certain brain functions affecting your
concentration and co-ordination. Too much alcohol can affect your
speech, memory and judgement, and increases your chance of having an
accident.

Accidents

Drinking increases your chance of an accident at home, at work and on
the roads. About a third of all domestic accidents, nearly 40 per cent of
deaths in fires, and a quarter of deaths from drowning are related to
heavy drinking. Drinking and driving has long been known to be linked
with road accidents. About one-sixth of all road deaths are caused by
drink/driving (around 700 deaths in 1991). Nearly a third of deaths

among women between 15 to 24 years are owing to accidents, particularly road accidents, and alcohol is a factor. Less well known is that an estimated 30 per cent of pedestrians involved in fatal road traffic accidents have drunk more alcohol than the legal limit for driving.

Nutrition problems

Alcohol is high in calories, so if you are watching your weight, cutting down on alcohol will help. Some drinkers substitute alcohol for food, which can lead to vitamin and other deficiencies, since alcohol doesn't contain much in the way of nutrition.

Sexual health

Excess alcohol seems to damage the immune system, which is a particular problem if you are HIV positive. Alcohol consumption may also influence sexual behaviour, removing inhibitions and judgement and increasing risk-taking. Casual sexual relationships are more likely to occur under the influence of alcohol, and safer sex is less likely to be practised. This increases the risk of sexually transmitted diseases, including HIV.

Trying for a baby or pregnant

If you're trying to get pregnant, it is a good idea for both you and your partner to cut down the amount of alcohol you drink. Drinking above the recommended weekly limits may reduce both your own and your partner's fertility. And the most vulnerable time for the development of the foetus is in the early weeks after conception, before you even know you are pregnant.

Once you are pregnant, alcohol can pass easily from you to your baby through the placenta. Many women decide to give up alcohol altogether during pregnancy, because they are worried about possible harm to the baby, or because they simply go off it, especially during the early months when they may feel a bit queasy. If you choose not to cut out alcohol altogether, then limiting yourself to one or two units once or twice a week will minimise any risk.

Studies have shown that even moderate drinking (more than 10 units a week) may be harmful to the foetus, being associated with congenital abnormalities, higher incidence of stillbirths, growth retardation, and delayed physical and mental development. Binge drinking (5 or 6 units on one occasion) is also harmful. And heavy alcohol consumption (more than 8 units a day) during pregnancy can result in a child being born with Foetal Alcohol Syndrome. The baby is born with facial and physical deformities, and may be mentally retarded and slow to grow and develop.

If you are breast feeding

Alcohol is passed to your baby in small quantities in breast milk, which may affect the baby's sleeping, feeding or bowels. If you've had several drinks, it's best to wait a while to allow your body to get rid of the alcohol before breast feeding. On average, it takes one hour for the body to get rid of one unit of alcohol.

How to be a sensible drinker

Although most people are aware that alcohol can affect health, most of us are not particularly concerned about our own drinking habits. Women are much more likely to identify smoking, stress, exercise, safer sex or weight problems as important for their health. Men are twice as likely as women to claim to have tried to reduce the amount of alcohol they drink. But making sure you're sensible about your drinking can be another way of improving your health. You may find the following suggestions helpful when thinking about your drinking. You don't have to follow them all, work out what's best for you:

- work out how much you're drinking by keeping a drinking diary for a week.

- if you're drinking more than the recommended limit of 14 units, you can use the diary to work out when, where and with whom you drink most. This may help you decide how to cut down.

- try to keep one or two drink-free days each week.

- choose low-alcohol or alcohol-free drinks instead of alcohol sometimes. As well as cutting down on alcohol, they can help to control weight, and some people prefer them. Most low-alcohol lagers are about one-third the strength of ordinary lagers.

- sip your drink more slowly and drink smaller measures. Don't try to keep up with other drinkers.

- never drink if you're going to drive or use machinery.

- avoid drinking if you're taking other drugs, always check with your doctor or pharmacist.

- ask yourself why you're having a drink. It may help you to decide not to. Make drinking a conscious choice rather than a habit.

- find enjoyable ways to socialise or relax which doesn't necessarily involve drinking alcohol.

- if you're finding it hard to cut down, you can get help (see below).

Do you have a drink problem?

It's sometimes hard to know if you are drinking because of problems, or if your drinking is causing the problems. Finances, relationships, health, employment or other areas of your life may all be affected because of your drinking. You may have a problem because of someone else's drinking. Alcohol is responsible for a great deal of marital conflict including communication problems and domestic violence.

Not everyone with a drink problem has to give up drinking altogether.

You may be able to find a way to drink more sensibly having tackled the underlying problems first. Think about situations that trigger your drinking. Use the drink diary to see if there are certain places where you drink more – at home on your own, in certain clubs and bars, with certain friends. Do you drink to help cope with feelings or escape from worries, as a temporary relief from stress and anxiety, or to help you relax? Do you drink instead of expressing feelings of anger or frustration, or after a row at home or work.

If any of these are true for you, you can try some of the suggestions for sensible drinking above. It may help to try to build up other ways of coping in these situations. You could learn some relaxation skills (see page 31), try to think more positively about yourself, talk with a friend, or seek professional counselling.

Getting help

There is certainly still a social stigma attached to women drinking. Both problem drinking and drunkenness in men is much more tolerated. Dependency on alcohol in women may interfere with their expected roles as partners, mothers and workers, and is therefore considered unacceptable. Women may fear being seen as unfit to care for their children. It's easy to feel you are a failure, and keep your drink problems to yourself as a guilty secret. Acknowledging that you have a problem may be the most important step to getting help.

Your doctor can provide help or refer you to other agencies, such as local councils on alcohol or alcohol problem advisory services, or may be able to offer counselling and support. Alcoholics Anonymous offers support and self-help groups across the UK for problem drinkers and their families.

Alcohol Treatment Services may offer a range of different approaches to treatment including detoxification and group therapy. Unfortunately, services are sometimes not particularly sensitive to women's needs, especially related to childcare and the need to have a choice about mixed or women-only groups.

Are you the right weight for your height?

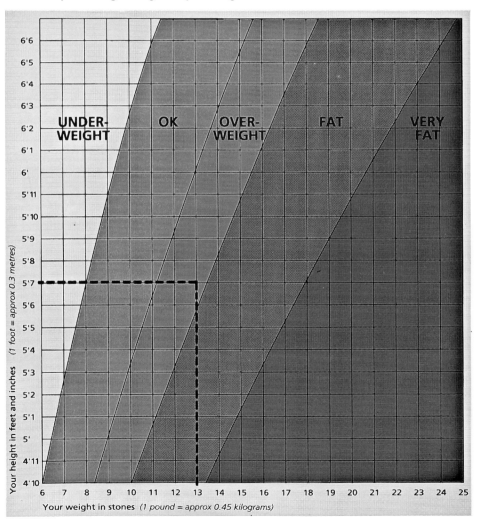

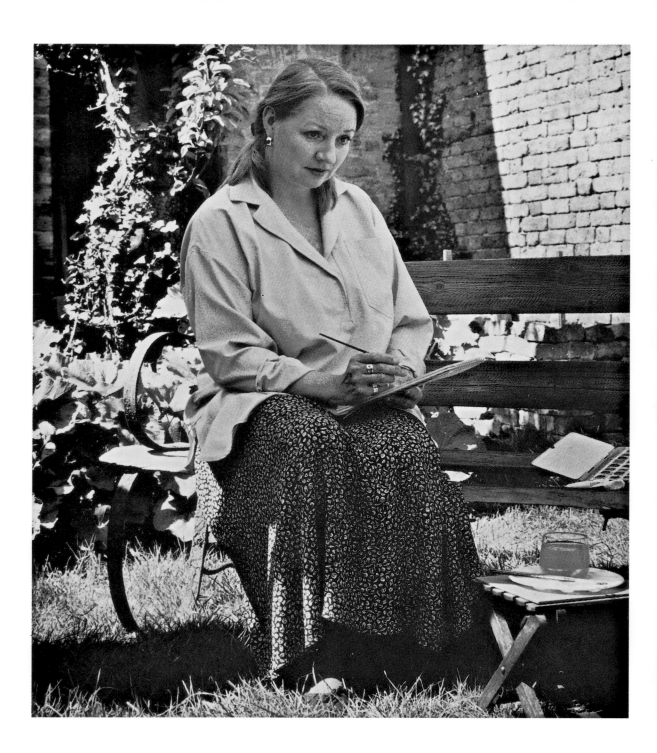

This chapter covers some common themes around mid-life, and issues that you may face as you grow older. Other chapters cover a variety of topics that may also be of interest or relevance to you. Everyone has a different experience of growing older. But whether you are with a partner or alone, have children or not, are in paid work, full- or part-time, live close to an extended family or not, what characterises mid-life for us all is the need to confront and deal with change.

The feeling that you are growing old may be related to events – the menopause, children leaving home, retirement – or to chronological age. Very often we do not consider ourselves to be old until faced with illness or dependency, when we can no longer get about and do the things we have always done. For some women, the approach of their 40th birthday is enough to send them into a state of high anxiety. Society does not paint a favourable picture of older women – it is very unusual to see positive images portrayed in the media, and much of the language used to describe them reflects negative attitudes.

People, especially women, are living longer. Women are a dis-proportionately large percentage of the elderly population. If you take retirement to be the start of 'old age' many women can look forward to two or more decades of active independent life beyond that, and at different stages will have different needs and interests. On the plus side, you may have more time to spend on yourself; you may feel freer to do what you want and to say what you think (perhaps not caring as much about what other people think). You may have more self-confidence, perhaps even more money.

For many women, mid- and later life will be characterised by active independence, when you can enjoy good health and have the time to pursue your own needs and interests. Women bring a wealth of experience and skills to this stage, are supportive of others as carers within the family, as workers and volunteers, and have time and willingness to develop in new directions and try new things. Many of us will also face a number of events and health problems that are a common part of growing older. Some are easier to deal with or cope with than others. All of them require good information, and appropriate support and care. This chapter considers some of the common situations facing you in mid-life and considers what you can do to help yourself and where you can go for help.

Menopause

Your experience of the menopause will depend a lot on your particular circumstances – how you feel about the idea of the menopause and how prepared you are for it. You may view this time as full of rewards and opportunities; it can mean freedom from using contraception; more time for yourself; or you may feel distressed by the signals that you are reaching the end of your fertile years, or just growing older.

What is the menopause?

Menopause is the process of the ending of menstruation. It is a natural event which every woman experiences if she lives long enough. It occurs when your level of hormone production, which has been slowly declining, drops too low to maintain the menstrual cycle and the ovaries stop releasing eggs. Hormone levels fluctuate during the menopause, often producing very unpredictable periods and other symptoms. After the menopause you continue to produce female hormones such as oestrogen, but at much lower levels.

When will it happen?

For most women the menopause takes place between the ages of 45 and 55, but it may happen earlier or later. There does not seem to be any connection between the age of starting periods and the onset of the menopause. The length of the menopause also varies. For some women, periods end abruptly, others go through a stage of irregular periods when the amount of bleeding is changeable. This may last for anything from a few months to several years and can be frustrating, especially if the possibility of pregnancy adds to the uncertainty. Having your ovaries removed before reaching the menopause induces an early and accelerated menopause, unless you are given hormone replacement therapy.

What are the signs?

The changes that you may experience during the menopause are caused by changing levels of hormones in your blood stream. Not every woman is affected, and there are different degrees of severity. The most common signs are:

- irregular and unpredictable periods, sometimes with increased pre-menstrual syndrome
- hot flushes
- vaginal dryness
- osteoporosis (a common process of ageing, sometimes accelerated during the menopause).

Premenstrual syndrome (PMS)

If you are generally affected by PMS it may become prolonged when periods are delayed or missed during the menopause. Hormone levels which are too low to start a period can still produce premenstrual symptoms (see page 48).

Hot flushes

A hot flush is a wave of heat passing over the body, sometimes accompanied by redness, sweating or tingling. Hot flushes at night are sometimes called night sweats. Chills often follow hot flushes. The frequency and intensity of flushes and sweats vary enormously – some women never experience them, others have flushes occasionally, while a minority of women feel their lives are disrupted by flushes.

Hot flushes are not as obvious to everyone else as to you, and for many women the anxiety about having a flush in a public place is worse than the flush itself. Because hot flushes are an outward sign of the menopause, they may be especially hard to deal with if you are worried about work colleagues or friends knowing you are going through the menopause. It may help to let them know, so that they understand your situation.

The treatment usually offered by doctors for hot flushes and other menopausal symptoms is hormone replacement therapy (HRT). There are some possible side-effects and it is important to have enough information to make an informed decision (see page 272).

Vaginal lubrication

Most but not all women experience some degree of vaginal dryness during the menopause and sometimes this can cause problems. The vagina needs lubrication to cleanse itself and fight infection – vaginal dryness can make you prone to vaginal and urinary infections (see section on Extra help, page 269).

After the menopause, vaginal secretion is decreased in most women. This may make penetration painful and difficult, but other forms of sexual or sensual activity can ease the dryness by increasing vaginal lubrication.

Osteoporosis

Women are at far greater risk of osteoporosis than men because, as the menopause approaches, the level of the hormone oestrogen declines, slowing down calcium absorption and speeding up the loss of bone mass.

Osteoporosis is a disease of the bones, in which they become too porous so that they break easily. It affects more than one woman in four, compared with one man in twenty. The condition develops silently over many years, gradually and without discomfort. It usually shows up after the age of 50, but may start as early as the late thirties. You may become aware of it suddenly, with a painful fracture after only a slight fall or awkward movement, or your clothes may appear not to fit any more because your spine is starting to curve.

Factors which may increase the risk of osteoporosis include:

- early menopause (naturally or after hysterectomy) before 45 years
- prolonged loss of periods (e.g. from anorexia or bulimia nervosa)
- family history of osteoporosis
- low calcium intake or absorption
- lack of exercise
- smoking

What you can do to help yourself

There are a number of ways you can help yourself to have a more comfortable menopause – including making changes in your life, exercise, diet, and natural remedies. The following ideas are not a 'prescription' for a healthy menopause, merely some suggestions you may like to try.

Look after yourself

- Put your own needs first for a change, making time to relax or follow your own interests.
- Try to identify and reduce stress in your life (see section on Stress, pages 17-23).

- Take some regular exercise e.g. swimming, yoga, dancing, keep-fit classes or walking (see pages 194-197). Eat a balanced diet with as much fresh fruit and vegetables as you can afford (see pages 215-217). Make sure you get enough calcium (see Osteoporosis, pages 266-267).
- Start something new just for yourself – learn a skill you've always wanted to, join a class or group, begin a new hobby or interest, or take up one you have dropped because of other commitments.
- Strengthen the relationships and friendships that are important to you, and be open to making new friends (see page 2).

Unpredictable periods

- Keep track of any changing patterns in your periods by keeping a diary to show the timing and length of each period.
- If you experience pre-menstrual syndrome (PMS), note it in the diary so that you can see if it follows any pattern and you will know when to expect it even when your periods have stopped.
- Remember to continue using contraception as you might get pregnant for at least 18 months after your last period.

Hot flushes and night sweats

- Try to cut down on cigarettes and sugar (these can cause sweating and flushes in people not having the menopause), alcohol, tea and coffee (see Ideas for reducing stress, pages 21-23).
- Check with your doctor if any drugs you are taking could be making your flushes worse.
- Tell your family and friends what hot flushes are and how you feel when you have them. Explain that at times you may need to switch heating off or on and that you expect them to understand.
- Ensure you are able to adjust your temperature, if you need to, by dressing in easily removed layers, and sleeping with the bedding loose.
- Avoid artificial fibres (e.g. nylon) for your clothes and bedding as they

increase sweating. Wear natural fibres as much as possible (cotton or wool, or mixtures with some natural fibres in them) and use cotton sheets.

- When you feel a hot flush coming on, don't fight it, just let it wash over you. Try to relax with some deep breathing (see pages 34-37).
- Place the insides of your wrists and arms on a cold surface or under running water during a flush or sweat.
- Keep a change of night clothes and bedding and some talcum powder or cologne handy in case of a severe night sweat. You will get back to sleep more quickly if you feel comfortable.

Extra help

- Pelvic floor exercises can increase the suppleness and elasticity of the vagina and other internal organs (see pages 278-280).
- More imaginative and tender love-making, or masturbation, will increase vaginal secretions and reduce the likelihood of infections.
- A cream or jelly may help. There are several available, e.g. Aci-jel is a jelly which is slightly acid to restore the vagina to its natural acidic balance and so prevent infection. It's available over the counter from your chemist. KY jelly is a simple lubricant which may be used to help penetrative sex be more comfortable. Hormone creams are available on prescription and HRT restores natural vaginal secretions.

Making changes

To prevent osteoporosis you need to keep active and have a balanced diet from early adulthood onwards. But it is never too late to make some changes:

- Eat plenty of foods rich in calcium, particularly milk, cheese, and yoghurt. Low-fat versions have just as much calcium. Other good sources include nuts, canned fish and dark green leafy vegetables such as broccoli.
- Keep active – bones need steady regular exercise to help make them

strong and reduce bone loss. It's best to do a little steady exercise every day. Brisk walking, keep-fit classes, running, dancing, cycling, or using stairs are all good examples. While swimming is good general exercise, it does not exercise bones or prevent bone loss because the weight of your body is supported by the water.

- Avoid smoking – smoking accelerates the onset of the menopause by two to five years, and may suppress new bone growth. Passive smoking (see pages 250-251) can also have a bad effect on bones.

Getting help

You may feel you need more help with the symptoms you are experiencing during the menopause, and want to talk things through with your doctor. Some symptoms, like very heavy periods, bleeding between periods or any other irregularities, should always be investigated by a doctor. Many women go at some point to their doctor for advice about the menopause. Symptoms such as PMS, tiredness, depression or aches and pains may be dismissed too easily, perhaps with a prescription for sleeping pills or tranquillisers without any real investigation into the problem. Other symptoms, such as hot flushes, are more likely to be taken seriously. Often the treatment offered is hormone replacement therapy (HRT), but there is sometimes little opportunity provided to talk through the advantages and risks and look at some of the issues involved (see pages 271-273). Doctors do not always make it clear why HRT is being prescribed, some women believing that they have been given hormone treatment to help them sleep or 'cope'. Others may not even be told that they are being given hormones at all, or doctors may fail to offer HRT because they do not recognise the value of it.

"You need someone to talk to and describe what you are going through. You want reassurance – knowing that nothing is wrong can make you feel better. And you want above all the chance to think through different options."

'My doctor told me I needed HRT. He didn't give me any explanation about possible side-effects, and I felt too nervous to ask, as if I was questioning his judgement'.

Of course, not all doctors are unhelpful about the menopause. If you feel dissatisfied with your first encounter, it is possible to ask to see another doctor in your practice, or to consider changing doctors (see pages 297-299). It may be possible to attend a Well-Women Clinic or Menopause Clinic. These may be few and far between. They are sometimes part of the NHS, or may be run by voluntary organisations. They are often very informal and 'woman-centred', listening to what women say about their own experiences and offering a range of treatments and remedies, including complimentary therapies. To find out about clinics near you ask your GP, Community Health Council, or Citizens' Advice Bureau.

Hormone replacement therapy

Hormone replacement therapy (HRT) is based on the idea that, as you produce less oestrogen and progesterone at the menopause, it should be possible to replace the lost hormones, thereby avoiding the changes which might take place as the body adjusts to lowered levels of naturally produced hormones.

HRT has a real place in helping some women with specific problems around the menopause, particularly if you are at high risk of osteoporosis or heart disease. But it is important that you know the risks as well as the advantages, so that you can make an informed choice, and it should be prescribed only after careful assessment, and monitored through regular medical checks.

What HRT can do

HRT is used to treat symptoms of menopause with oestrogen and progestogen, or oestrogen alone when a women has had a hysterectomy. Treatment may be in the form of pills, skin patches, creams, or implants under the skin. In particular it may be used to:

- relieve such short-term menopausal symptoms as hot flushes, sweats and vaginal dryness
- help prevent osteoporosis, although it cannot reverse the process of bone loss, and cannot replace bone if the osteoporosis is advanced
- reduce the long-term risks of heart attacks and stroke
- relieve the after-effects of hysterectomy and removal of ovaries.

HRT may also help with depression, insomnia (by reducing the disturbing effects of night sweats and hot flushes), and migraine. It may also restore self-confidence and libido by helping with vaginal lubrication. It can increase fluid retention and so 'puff' out the skin and reduce wrinkle lines. Because of these effects HRT has sometimes been described as having 'rejuvenating' powers.

Side-effects of HRT

- You will have a monthly bleed, like a light period, if you have not had a hysterectomy.
- You may find that you experience breast tenderness, weight gain, and other premenstrual-syndrome-type symptoms. These symptoms should disappear after the first two months and, if not, the dose or type of HRT should be changed.
- There is the possible increased risk of breast cancer when taken for ten years or more.

Deciding about HRT

It's important to talk through all the possibilities with your doctor before coming to a decision about HRT.

You may decide it is appropriate for you if:

- you have had ovaries and womb removed before the menopause (especially before 45 years). Women who have had their ovaries removed are particularly at risk from osteoporosis
- you are suffering from osteoporosis, and want to reduce further bone loss
- you have a family history of osteoporosis
- you have a high risk of osteoporosis detected by bone scan
- you have a history of loss of periods (e.g. through anorexia or bulimia nervosa)

HRT may not be appropriate for you if any of the following apply:

- you have a history of oestrogen-dependent tumours of genital tract or breast
- you have a family history of breast cancer
- you have undiagnosed irregular bleeding
- you are pregnant
- you have uncontrolled hypertension (high blood pressure)
- you have fibroids
- you have endometriosis
- you have had recent thrombo-embolic disease

Before starting HRT

If you want to consider using HRT, find a doctor who will explain all the different advantages and risks to you and who will help you choose the preparation which will provide an effective dose with the fewest risks.

- Before starting HRT your doctor should give you an internal examination of the uterus and cervix, a blood pressure check, breast examination and urine tests. She should also find out about your health up to now, and family health. Find out what future medical checks you will need, and how often these should be done.
- Find out what checks to do for yourself — for example, checking your breasts each month (after your period if you are taking both oestrogen and progestogen).

- Discuss what type of hormone preparation you will need. Most commonly it will be in tablet form. However, some oestrogens are available as implants which are put under the skin. There are also creams containing oestrogen and these are sometimes prescribed to help vaginal dryness.
- Check with your doctor whether you will have bleeding.
- Find out about any side-effects that need reporting, for example, any irregular bleeding. Agree when you should return to see the doctor.
- Discuss how long you should take the hormone treatment.

Hysterectomy

Many women find it is quite difficult to come to terms with a hysterectomy. Many of us feel that even if we have passed through our menopause many years before our womb is bound up with our womanhood. For some women, a hysterectomy may have a particularly devastating effect as it ends all hopes of future motherhood. Post-menopausal women find it easier to come to terms with hysterectomy than younger women.

In all cases hysterectomy should be seen as a treatment of 'last resort', and the implications of the operation should be carefully explained by your doctor. Many doctors and gynaecologists believe that an unnecessary number are carried out, and in some areas of the world hysterectomies are so common that it seems as though doctors need a reason not to operate rather than a good reason to treat. In the USA, hysterectomy is particularly common and some surgeons even advocate routine hysterectomy when childbearing is over to prevent risk of cancer. British doctors are rather less scalpel-happy.

Hysterectomy is a major operation which usually requires about a week in hospital, followed by a fairly lengthy recuperation period. The exact recovery time will depend on the woman's age and general fitness, but it is often six weeks or so before she can return to her normal activities. In some cases, when the operation is technically difficult, e.g. large fibroids, a mid-line cut is used. More often a bikini-line cut is used, which leaves a small, neat scar. An alternative approach is through the vagina (vaginal hysterectomy), which leaves no external scar at all. New techniques including 'keyhole' (laparoscopic) hysterectomy and laser hysterectomy, where only the womb lining is removed, are becoming more widely available. Your surgeon will advise you which is most suitable for you.

A *total hysterectomy* involves the surgical removal of the uterus and cervix, a *subtotal or partial hysterectomy* leaves the cervix intact. Usually a hysterectomy does not involve the removal of the fallopian tubes or the ovaries, which means that it does not trigger the menopause. It does, however, bring a woman's fertile life to a close and it puts an end to periods. Although removing the womb doesn't cause menopause if the ovaries are left, many women do go through an early menopause following a hysterectomy. It is important to be aware of this, as you might need to consider HRT.

A hysterectomy will almost definitely be recommended when a woman suffers from:

- severe, uncontrollable uterine bleeding
- a very severe and uncontrollable pelvic infection
- a cancerous growth in the vagina, cervix or uterus which does not respond to other treatment.

A hysterectomy may also be essential as part of surgery necessary to deal with a life-threatening disorder elsewhere in the abdominal cavity — for example, in the intestines or bladder. In rare cases it may be impossible to deal with the problem without first removing the uterus.

Sometimes hysterectomy is recommended when a woman suffers from a severe form of one of the following conditions:

- painful, recurrent attacks of pelvic inflammatory disease (see pages 116-117)
- extensive endometriosis which does not respond to other treatments, especially when the condition is so severe as to leave the woman infertile, or when she has completed her family
- uterine fibroids (which have not responded to other less extreme forms of treatment)

Studies show that women who have had hysterectomies are more likely to suffer from depression than those who have not, especially if they are under 40 when the operation takes place. This is far more likely to be a consequence of the emotional impact of the operation than the physical impact. However, if your doctor recommends a hysterectomy it is worth getting a second opinion just to ensure it is absolutely necessary. Other new methods of treatment are being developed to deal with fibroids, tumours and some cervical conditions for which hysterectomy was once routine.

If you face a possible hysterectomy it is important to remember the following:

- Hysterectomy will not affect your enjoyment of sex or make you less sexually desirable.
- The presence or absence of your uterus does not physically affect your sexual feelings, nor the way in which you are aroused nor the way you feel to your partner. The only effect it may have is a psychological one. If you are feeling depressed, worried and insecure you are unlikely to enjoy sex. Communication is the key to any difficulties. Share any fears you may have with your partner. Do not hesitate to raise any concerns, no matter how trivial you think they may seem, with your doctor.
- Hysterectomy will not make you fat.
- Some women do put on weight after a hysterectomy but this is owing to the prolonged period of rest needed after the operation. If you are immobile you will burn up fewer calories, so, unless you eat less, you are bound to put on a little weight. When you are fit and active again, you will probably find that the pounds fall away – especially if you eat sensibly and exercise regularly.
- If you have been operated on by a good and skilful gynaecologist, and the surgery is successful, the only after-effects of a hysterectomy should be that you have no more periods and you cannot possibly conceive. You might think that this adds to your quality of life rather than detracts from it.

Incontinence

It is estimated that between 2 and 3 million people in the UK suffer from incontinence. A large percentage is over 65, but certain types of incontinence are not uncommon in much younger women. Incontinence is not inevitable, and it is worth getting help early for the problem, however embarrassing it may seem.

A common problem for many women is what is known as 'stress incontinence'. A slight leak of urine occurs when you cough, sneeze, laugh or exert yourself during strenuous activity. It is caused by a deterioration in the muscles and tissues in the pelvic area. Lack of exercise, or exercise of the wrong sort, or perhaps childbirth, has allowed the muscles to become stretched and to lose their elasticity. It may also be related to changes during the menopause – the vaginal lining may become dry and sore and this can affect the bladder and urethra (the tube which urine passes through), making you feel as if you need to keep passing urine.

What you can do for yourself?

It is important to get professional help for incontinence as soon as possible but there are also things you can do for yourself to improve your condition and overall feeling of well-being.

Think about:

your diet   •   A healthy diet high in fibre will help prevent constipation which can cause both bladder and bowel problems. Keeping to a healthy weight by staying active and avoiding overeating can also help prevent stress incontinence.

fluid intake   •   You may think that restricting the amount you drink will help your bladder control, but in fact the opposite is true. Drinking plenty of fluid each day helps the kidneys to function properly and prevents urine from being too concentrated. You need between six and nine cups each day.

pelvic floor exercises   •   Simple exercises to help you control your pelvic muscles and improve their strength may be all you need to become continent. It may be a few weeks before you notice any improvement, so keep doing the exercises every day. Once you get in practice you can do them anywhere at any time without anyone knowing.

Pelvic floor exercises

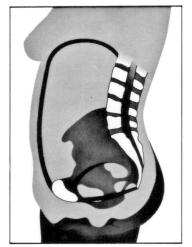

diagram (a)

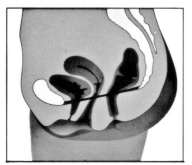

diagram (b)

The pelvic floor consists of layers of muscle stretching like a hammock from the pubic bone (in front) to the end of the backbone (see diagram a). These muscles hold the bladder, uterus and bowel in place.

Muscle fibres circle the three openings (urethra, vagina and anus) forming sphincters which act like valves. The urinary sphincter stops and starts the flow of urine.

A healthy active pelvic floor has a normal firmness which responds to stretch and movement. The muscle floor is a firm supportive hammock forming a straight line from the pubic bone to the end of the backbone (see diagram b). The muscles are always slightly tense and the sphincters are normally closed.

Weakness or injury, owing to lack of exercise, childbirth, or ageing, causes the pelvic floor to sag (see diagram c). This can result in loose vaginal walls, prolapse of the uterus, constipation, incomplete emptying of the bladder, leaking of urine under pressure (for example, when coughing, sneezing or laughing) and other problems.

If you suffer from stress incontinence, then your control *can* improve. If

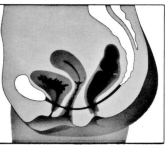
diagram (c)

you have trouble reaching the loo first thing in the morning, it will help to do a few pelvic floor exercises before you stand up. If after practising the following exercises for a month or so, your symptoms do not improve, go to your doctor.

The exercises may also be helpful in improving your sex life, and helping your body cope with the physical demands of pregnancy.

How to do pelvic floor exercises

These exercises involve lifting up the pelvic floor and tightening the sphincters. To identify the muscles you are trying to strengthen, imagine yourself stopping the urine flow, and concentrate on the muscles you are using. A good test of muscle strength is to see if you can actually slow down or stop the urine flow.

You can feel the pelvic floor muscles working by placing one or two fingers in your vagina and tensing. You could try this during sex, and get feedback and encouragement from your partner.

Start by lying down so there is less pressure on the pelvic floor from the weight of the pelvic organs. If you cannot feel the muscles working in this position, raise your bottom on a pillow. The pelvic floor will sink into your body, closer to the position you are trying to achieve. As you progress you will be able to do the exercises standing or sitting.

Each of these exercises will strengthen the pelvic floor. You can choose one or use a combination. It is important not to strain or overwork your pelvic floor, so keep to no more than 50 contractions a day.

Exercise One
- Contract or draw up your pelvic floor, hold for three seconds, relax and repeat five times. Continue this during the day building up to ten groups of five contractions. Overworking this muscle may result in soreness. If this

happens, reduce the number you do or stop the exercises for a few days, and then gradually increase again.

Exercise Two •   Imagine you are in a lift, and as you go up, try to draw in the muscles gradually. When you reach your limit, don't just let go; you must go down floor by floor, gradually relaxing the muscles in stages. When you reach the basement, let go of all the tension and release. Then come back up to the ground floor so the pelvic floor is slightly tense and able to hold the pelvic organs in place.

Exercise Three •   Raise the entire pelvic area as though sucking water into the vagina. Relax and repeat five times. You can insert a finger and feel the vagina drawing in. This series of five contractions may be repeated four to six times a day building up to 20 to 30 contractions a day.

Getting help

You may be feeling embarrassed about your problem and unsure about how to go about getting help. In fact incontinence is a very common problem and your GP will be happy to discuss it with you. If you prefer, you could talk to a community nurse or health visitor – you can phone your GP's surgery or health centre and ask to speak to either of them.

Think about:

who to talk to •   the important thing is to find someone who makes you feel at ease, and takes your problem seriously. If the first person you ask is not very helpful, don't be discouraged.

some questions you may be asked •   about your general health and whether you are taking any medicines and about your bladder control. How many times do you pass water each day? Do you ever not make it to the loo in time? Do you leak when you cough, laugh or run? Do you have any trouble actually passing water? Do you ever dribble after you have passed water? Is the bed ever wet in the morning?

keeping a record • you could keep a simple chart for a few days which shows when you passed water, the time of day when you are wet and whether you needed to change your clothes, the number of drinks you have, etc.

Treatment you may be offered

If your problem is severe or has been going on for a long time, you will probably need some treatment in addition to any self-help. Your doctor will help you decide what is most appropriate for your needs – including pelvic floor exercises, retraining the bladder, medication, and, in a few cases, surgery.

Time for Yourself

Growing older will almost certainly bring about changes in the way you use your time. When faced with the frantic demands of dependent children, full- or part-time paid work and a home to organise, the thought of free time may seem like some distant illusion. Your partner, too, may be at a stage with the least time and energy to give, while making many demands on you.

As children grow more independent, they may leave a gap that needs filling with new commitments and activities. Work commitments may also reduce as you get older – you may want to devote less time to building a career or putting in long hours, or decide to take on less demanding roles. Redundancy or retirement leave a space previously taken by paid work. This new freedom can offer enormous scope for taking up fresh interests or developing in different directions. But the very demands that have exercised you up to now make it likely that you have had little practice or experience along the way of using time for yourself. Men are much more likely to have found time to pursue their own interests outside work hours, which makes them better prepared when it comes to children leaving home or employment ending.

Reaching mid-life may leave some women feeling lonely, bored or isolated. It may take some time to adjust to a new situation where your roles are changing, leaving you feeling less sure that you are valued and needed. Such feelings of self-doubt may stem from experiences over the years where your confidence has been undermined and you have been led to doubt your own worth. By thinking of all the coping strategies you have had to develop to survive up to now, you will begin to realise you have enormous strengths and lots of useful experiences to build on.

Making the most of opportunities

Doing your own thing

Think about the things you have always wanted to do but so far haven't had the chance to pursue. What stopped you up to now? How could you begin to take them up? What are the barriers? And how can you overcome these?

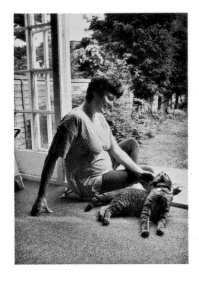

In order to find out about local opportunities and activities on offer, you can contact your local council, adult education centre, leisure centre, your library, local council or voluntary service or Citizens' Advice Bureau. Local radio may be a good source of information, too, and building on your existing networks such as the church, local groups, or tenants' association, can be a good way of seeking out new opportunities.

Don't be afraid of what your friends or family may say or think. Children in particular may be good at pouring scorn on things which they see as 'unsuitable', 'unsafe' or plain embarrassing. Remind them of the way you support them in doing their own thing, and tell them to mind their own business! Partners may become uncomfortable if you start getting your life together and become more independent. Elderly parents may fear they will get less attention if their daughter takes up interests of her own. We have our own perceptions about what we can and cannot do, and what is appropriate, which might discourage us from pursuing some leisure or education opportunities. Most of us are very good at finding reasons for not doing things. Be aware of the reasons or excuses you often use, and think through counter-arguments and ways to get round any obstacles you may put in your own way.

Taking up education or training

Many women in mid-life opt for some kind of education, either to improve qualifications, to follow a particular interest or as a way of getting back to work. Think about the things you are good at. Many women find this very difficult and tend to underestimate and devalue their skills. You may lack confidence about starting or returning to study, fearing you are out of touch, too stupid or too old. But if you take the time to think through the staggering number of skills it takes to run a home, bring up children, manage a family budget, take care of sick members of the family, hold down a job, often all at the same time, then it becomes clearer that you do have an enormous amount to offer. This can increase your confidence, and give you an idea of what direction to go in.

Nowadays, people of all ages study, and many courses welcome 'mature' students because of the depth of experience they bring to a course. Some courses are specially designed for women returners. Many women taking up study in mid-life have found that age is not a barrier to learning, and that the breadth of experience and knowledge they have is a great advantage.

You may need to be persistent to find your way around the variety of courses and classes on offer. Try contacting your local adult education institute, university extra-mural department, further education college, or library for information. If you live out of reach of colleges or adult education, you might investigate distance or correspondence learning.

One thing can lead to another. It isn't easy to make huge changes to your life straightaway. Instead, consider small steps you feel ready to take, and get support from those around you to try them out, maybe find a friend to accompany you. If your first attempts do not work out, don't be discouraged. If you start something and find you are not enjoying it, don't feel you have to carry on. There are lots more ways of using your time, and lots of different things to try out.

Thinking ahead to retirement

In the past, people spent most of their life working and did not survive long past retirement age. Nowadays, we may be free for many years to pursue our own interests. The traditional view that retirement is a time to decrease physical and mental activities is now questioned as research clearly shows the benefits of an active lifestyle. It is recognised that part of the decline experienced by some older people is owing to inactivity rather than to the ageing process.

Coping with change

If you think about how the world has changed during the lifetime of many older people today, you can see how skilful they have been at adapting.

Think about the changes you might be facing in the near and more distant future. There will be a whole spectrum, including: changes around work, social activities, free time, new relationships, children leaving home, new opportunities, grandchildren, parents dying, partner dying, where you live, illness and disability, becoming dependent on others. Some of these will be positive changes; others will be difficult to cope with or adjust to. It helps to recognise beforehand that you will be facing change, and that you have the skills and experience to cope with it.

Your strengths may include:
- coping and survival skills
- breadth of skills and experience
- previous experience of change
- adaptability
- time management skills
- friendships and supportive networks
- good health
- experience of relationships

One of the changes which many women face is a partner reaching retirement. This can have some far-reaching implications for them, not all of them positive. It's helpful to reflect on what effect your partner retiring may have on your life, and to consider the advantages and disadvantages of having a partner more often at home.

Acknowledging your feelings and discussing them with your partner may help. Think through what retirement will mean for you. In some ways, women never retire — we carry on cooking, cleaning, shopping and washing as we have always done, until we die or can do them no longer.

- Negotiate with your partner how tasks may be shared between you.
- Discuss how you can give each other the space you need to pursue your own separate interests after retirement.
- Plan ways that you can enjoy spending time together — for example, taking up a new hobby together, joining a club, going out together, seeing friends.

Caring for Others

Throughout their lives, many women take responsibility for caring for others – children, partners, grandchildren, and through the paid and voluntary work they do.

One of the situations that you may face as you grow older is the need to care for a partner, family member or friend as they become increasingly dependent through poor health or disability. Around 80 per cent of carers are women. While most carers want to care, many have gradually done more and for longer than they would have chosen. A variety of tasks may be involved – practical, such as shopping, cleaning, making meals, washing, dressing, toileting — and emotional, like keeping the people company, making them feel valued, and helping them face pain.

These responsibilities and commitments may take up 24 hours a day 7 days a week. Yet many women do not recognise themselves as carers, but see it as something they do if they care about, feel responsible for or are related to someone who needs help. This expectation is frequently shared by professionals and family members alike.

'When my mother suffered a severe stroke and was unable to continue living on her own independently, it was automatically assumed by both her GP and by my brother and his wife that I would have her to live with me. They reckoned that as I was living alone and worked only part-time it would not be too inconvenient! I can remember feeling invisible as practical arrangements were made with little reference to me. It wasn't that I didn't want to care – I just wanted to think through the options.'

'My daughter was coping on her own with a young child. Then she got the chance to go back to college, and asked me if I'd mind Yasmin each morning for her. I wanted to help out, but it felt like too big a commitment – I was on my own for the first time since having my own four children, and was looking forward to having time for myself. But it felt so selfish to say no.'

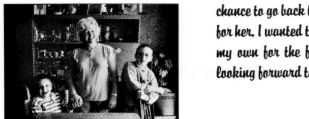

Considering taking on caring

It is very important to have the opportunity to think through implications before taking on caring for someone, and to explore all the possible options. If the caring role has developed gradually, decisions may have been made unnoticed. If a crisis intervenes, panic decisions may have been made under pressure from family members or health professionals.

Decisions made early on may have long-lasting and irreversible implications. It is important to feel you have made a choice about caring based on realistic information and an understanding of your own limits. For this you need:

- information about the way in which any illness or disability may develop in the future
- information about the back-up services available
- space to explore and acknowledge your own hopes and limits, what you feel able to do and what you are not prepared to do.

Think about:

- how much you are willing or able to undertake
- what changes it will make to your life, and whether you want this
- who else is affected (partner, children)
- how tasks could be shared and with whom
- what relevant services there are
- what alternatives there are to caring (sheltered accommodation, residential care, other).

Only when you have given yourself time to think through these questions and explore some of the possibilities can you be clear about what you can and cannot offer. Decisions may involve some compromises – not everyone involved may be able to achieve the ideal situation, but at least you will feel you have had some say in shaping what happens.

Coping with caring

If you are already caring for someone, you may experience ambivalent feelings about the situation – anger, frustration, hurt, resentment and guilt may co-exist with love, anxiety and concern for the person you are caring for.

Most women welcome 'professional' services which can ease your load, although they often seem quite peripheral compared to the caring tasks you are faced with and everything you have to do.

'If you're living with it, they just leave you to get on with it. They come and go if they come at all.'

'Every bit of help is welcome when you feel alone and overwhelmed with everything you have to do.'

But there are a bewildering number and range of services and organisations who may be able to help. You may have a range of needs, including financial needs; aids to help you with caring (for example, commodes, bath rails); support services such as meals on wheels, home helps, nursing services; and respite care.

As well as the practical help they can offer, these different agencies and workers can play an important part in making you feel valued and listened to, and your role recognised.

You may be working full- or part-time, or have given up work in order to care, especially if the person you are caring for is very dependent. Caring usually causes extra expense – in food, laundry and transport.

Caring for someone quite dependent at a distance (where you do not live with the person you are caring for) can have its own particular stresses. You may feel split between the needs of the person cared for, and the needs of your own family, if you have one. Your own needs are often entirely ignored. You may be resisting the pressure to have the person live with you or there may be pressures from your partner or children not to have them, leading to feelings of guilt.

'I was anxious that she would be ill and not able to call for help – she was always on my mind.'

'In a typical day I would telephone my dad first thing in the morning; visit him as soon as I'd taken the children to school, to get him washed and dressed; visit again with some supper late afternoon and help him back to bed; then telephone again last thing at night to make sure he was all right.'

There is often the need for reliable professional help in the case of distance caring. This can help overcome your feeling that you are not doing enough, and will help get over the problem of the person being alone and vulnerable.

'It's vital to be able to rely on regular back-up – you need to know someone is going in.'

Most carers experience deterioration in their own health after starting to look after someone who needs a lot of care. Stress, plus emotional and physical strain, are the main causes.

- Try to avoid conflict between your caring role and your partner, children or other family members by talking through with everyone what your boundaries are, and any difficulties you are facing in juggling all the demands made on you.
- Ask other family members to support you by helping out and sharing the responsibility.

- Acknowledge any feelings you may have of loss or grief, and give yourself time and space for these.
- Rather than feel guilty for not doing enough, recognise all the things you are doing.
- Make time for your own needs, your own self, your own life.

Getting help

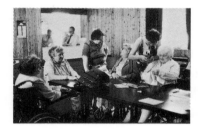

The range of services available to you as a carer will vary from place to place. Your District Health Authority and Social Services Department will both be able to help in a number of ways, and in addition there may be voluntary organisations in your area who can provide support and practical help. It's difficult to sort out exactly what you may be entitled to without some guidance – your GP, social services or Citizens' Advice Bureau may be able to give you some initial information, and point you in the right direction.

Respite care

- No one can go on and on without a break. You may be able to get a sitting-in service at home, or use a day centre, lunch club or day hospital care. For a longer break, there may be residential provision for the person you care for.

Financial help

- You may be entitled to a number of non-means-tested benefits, for example, attendance allowance, invalid care allowance, income supplement, help with transport.

Services and aids

- Services, including GPs, district nurses, community psychiatric nurses, health visitors, home helps or care assistants, meals on wheels.
- Aids and alterations to help with mobility, bathing, dressing, eating, lifting, incontinence equipment.
- Voluntary organisations like Age Concern, churches, befriending schemes, crossroads schemes may be able to help.

Ending caring

The end to caring is crucial. Whether the person you are caring for dies while still being cared for at home, or is moved to a hospital or residential care, it is important that you feel that you have achieved what you wanted, for as long as possible, and that your caring has been worth while. Give yourself time to adjust when the caring comes to an end; even if you have been caring for someone for a comparatively short time, you will need time to get used to the change. If the person you cared for has died, you will also be coming to terms with that loss and need to allow yourself to grieve.

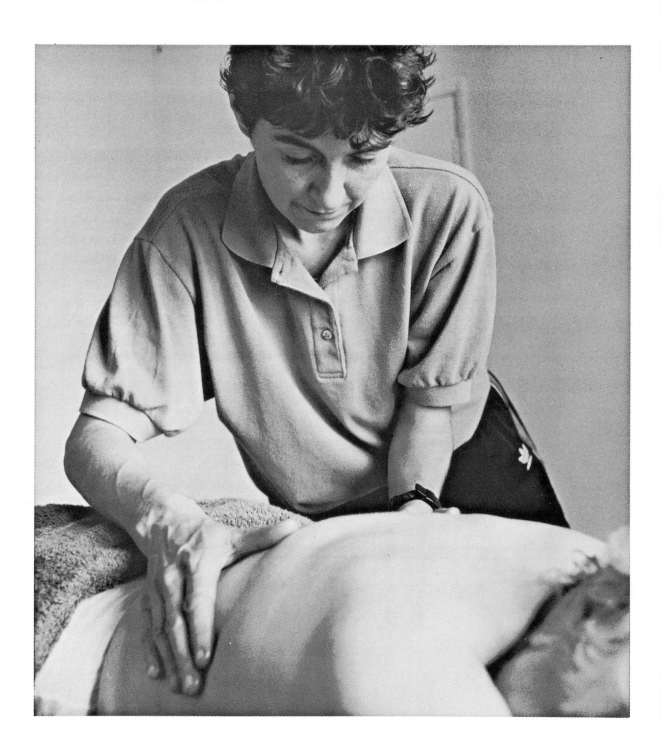

The Changing NHS

Most people agree that good health care should be available free to everyone at the time they need it. This is the principle on which the NHS was founded back in 1948, and it's valued just as highly today. But demands on health care resources keep on rising. Technological advances and growing medical expertise are making it possible to provide increasingly complex and expensive treatments. High-tech medical procedures such as hip replacements, organ transplants and kidney dialysis are costing the NHS more and more each year. Techniques such as in-vitro fertilisation, which are expensive and have a poor success rate, are only made available to a small number of women unless they can afford private treatment, thus creating a rationing system. Decisions about who should and should not get a certain treatment are fraught with difficulties, both for the individual doctors and patients concerned, and for society as a whole.

The NHS reforms which have been taking place over the last few years are requiring doctors to look very carefully at the range of procedures and treatments they offer, and weigh them up in terms of the 'health gain' derived from them. More and more emphasis is being placed on the ability of health care to 'add life to years' rather than just 'years to life'. And much more importance is being placed on 'preventive' health care – keeping us well in the first place, and picking up problems at an early stage when treatment may be simpler and more effective. For the first time ever, the UK has a national strategy for health, launched by the Government during 1992. Priorities have been identified and targets set for reducing illness and death in a number of key areas – cancer, sexual health, accidents, mental illness, and coronary heart disease. These particular health problems have been prioritised because they cause a large degree of illness and premature death, and because we know of ways to reduce or prevent them, both through individual action such as giving up smoking, and through government action, including safety legislation and national cancer screening programmes. These targets present a major challenge to the NHS, and to others who can influence health through social and environmental measures aimed at providing people with enough money and a safe and healthy environment in which to live and work.

What Women Want from Health Care

Women use the NHS more than men, especially during their reproductive years, when they consult doctors more than twice as often. Not only do we get ill more frequently, but we use doctors during the natural processes of pregnancy, childbirth and the menopause – which are commonly viewed as medical problems. Because some contraceptive methods carry a degree of risk to our health, they once again bring us into contact with health workers for check ups. We may take problems of infertility to a doctor too, sometimes leading to lengthy and highly technical medical treatments. Finally we are not only the main consumers of health care, but we're also the main providers, as nurses, and allied health workers of all kinds such as dieticians and physiotherapists, and as partners, mothers and daughters caring for other people in our lives and taking responsibility for their health.

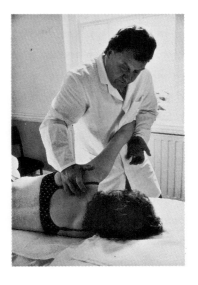

Women are fascinated by health. We spend much more time than men reading and finding out about it, and talking with our friends about our health problems. We are very open to new theories and ideas about health which the media regularly bombard us with, willing to try out new diets, allergy treatments, alternative therapies, or other innovations as we search for that elusive feeling of health and well-being. What we look for most of all is reliable and unbiased information which will help us understand what is going on in our bodies, and will give us a sense of control over our own health. We want to understand the treatments we are offered, what effects they may have on us, both good and bad, and what the alternatives are. Knowledge gives us the ability to make choices, and feel more in charge of our lives.

Sometimes the medical profession lets us down, not giving us the information we want, not taking our problems seriously or believing what we say. Their background and training does not always equip them to deal with the problems we bring. And the fact that most doctors are male can make it more difficult for them to understand the way we experience health problems.

Women are much more likely to be fobbed off with a prescription, or told to put up with symptoms. Doctors may make assumptions about us too, being quick to label us as anxious or depressed, without seeking out the real cause of our problems. And assumptions about our lifestyle can be particularly alienating. Many lesbians feel unable to tell their GP about their sexuality because of the way they fear they will be treated if they do. Instead, they may feel patronised or invisible.

'I went to my doctor with a rather bad vaginal discharge. He gave me some pessaries, and advised me to use condoms for the next couple of weeks when having sex. I didn't like to tell him I am a lesbian.'

What we really want is to be able to develop a relationship with the health professionals who care for us which allows us to play an active part in making decisions about our health, based on accurate information and a sound understanding on their part of who we are. Instead, we are often patronised with scanty explanations or over-directive advice based on false assumptions about us. Services need to be accessible too – easy for us to get to, at convenient times; and if we have to wait, then child-friendly areas make us feel much more welcome.

This chapter explores different settings within which health services are provided for women – through the NHS, voluntary organisations, and in the workplace; it considers some of the issues related to alternative health care and private health care; and it highlights a number of our rights as patients.

General Practitioners

Women and GPs

Your GP is the way in to almost all forms of medical care, both in the NHS and private. As a first port of call in most cases when you need health care or advice for yourself or someone you look after, a caring and competent GP can make the difference between good and indifferent medical care. Your GP may get to know you very well over a long period of time, and is probably the only health worker to have an idea of you as a whole person, rather than parts of a body that have gone wrong. His or her job is to help you keep well, by providing advice and preventive services such as immunisations, family planning and ante-natal care. Your GP will also be able to treat minor complaints and diagnose more serious problems, referring you to an appropriate specialist and following up on your progress.

In most cases your GP will look after the needs of the whole family, seeing you in your home context, which may be very relevant to any health problems you have. Caring for other members of the family, including children, partners or elderly parents, may bring you into frequent contact with your doctor. If you have children, you will usually be the one who takes them to the doctor for developmental checks, immunisation programmes, and when they are unwell. A survey carried out by the Women's National Commission found nearly one-third of women questioned had made their last medical consultation on behalf of someone else. Because you are likely to find yourself consulting your GP quite frequently, either for yourself or someone you care for, it is worth choosing one with care and developing a positive relationship which allows you to have the choice and control you require.

Choosing a GP practice

Everyone is entitled to have a GP. The choice is yours, provided the GP you choose is willing to accept you! Choosing the doctor who is going to look after your day-to-day health care needs some careful thought. One of the best ways to find a good doctor may be to talk to friends or neighbours to see who they recommend – make sure they are like-minded because not everyone looks for the same qualities from their doctor. If you don't come up with one this way, you'll find lists of GPs in main post offices and libraries, with the Family Health Service Authority (FHSA – look in the local phone book), Community Health Council, or Citizens' Advice Bureau. All GPs should produce a leaflet which details what services they offer, and this information may help you to narrow down the possible options before investigating further. Unfortunately, some rural areas may offer very little choice, in which case you may have to decide where you are going to compromise. If you can't find a GP to take you on, the FHSA will find you one.

Maybe you're looking for a GP because you have moved to a new area, or your GP has retired or died. You may be thinking about changing GP because you are not happy with the service you are getting. As with any other service, there will be some doctors who suit you and some who do not. Whatever your reason for finding a new GP, there are a number of points to think about before you make your choice:

- Is it a single or group practice? If single-handed, will you get on with the GP; and will you mind having to see a locum at times when your doctor is on holiday or ill?
- Does the practice include at least one woman GP? And, if so, is she so popular that it is very hard to get to see her?
- Is there an appointment system, or an open system where you just turn up and queue? Is it usually possible to see the GP of your choice at short notice, or are you likely to have to wait a few days for an appointment in

all but urgent cases?

- What are the surgery hours? Do they fit in with work and other commitments you may have?

- What range of services are offered by the practice (family planning services, smear tests, cholesterol testing, blood pressure clinics, antenatal care, child health clinics, well-women services, help with smoking cessation, and so on)? What about alternative practitioners, chiropodists, psychiatric nurses? These resources are more likely to be housed under one roof if the practice is based in a health centre.

- What is the practice policy on home visits? This may be especially important if you have young children, where a crisis can flare up quite quickly, often at night, or if you are caring for someone elderly who finds it hard to get to the surgery.

- Will you have the choice of a home birth if you want one? In what circumstances?

- What kind of relationship can you expect with your doctor? A positive, supportive consultation style has been shown to help patients get better more quickly, regardless of how much time the doctor spends with each patient.

- Does the practice hold its own funds? The NHS reforms have introduced this as an option for practices over a certain size. The implications are that your doctor may have more freedom to choose what treatment to offer and where to send you for treatment.

Having considered all these factors and decided on your priorities for a GP practice, you will need to match these up with what is on offer locally, probably making some compromises! Having narrowed the choice, try to arrange a visit to meet the doctor and get a general feel for the place. You will be able to see if there is up-to-date information available, if children are made welcome with books and toys, and what kind of attitude the receptionists have to patients, both face-to-face and on the 'phone. Once you are satisfied you have made a good choice you can apply to join the practice. Unfortunately, the really good practices tend to get filled quite quickly, so if this is the case you will need to find an alternative.

Some GPs are willing to accept patients on a private basis. While there are no lists of private GPs, you can ask if they are willing to treat you privately, or your local pharmacist may be able to advise you about who practises privately in your area.

Registering with a GP

People born in the UK are registered with a family doctor at birth and given a medical card. If you lose this, you can write to the Family Health Service Authority (FHSA), giving them details of your name, address, date of birth, and name and address of your last doctor. They will then issue a new one. If you've just taken up residence in the UK, you should find a GP to accept you on to their list, and they will then give you the necessary forms to register.

Having chosen a GP and been accepted by him or her, you should take your medical card to the surgery, and the receptionist will do the rest. While it is not necessary to discuss your decision or give a reason for wanting to change GP, it is common courtesy to let your existing doctor know. GPs are paid a fee for each patient on their list so records need to be kept up-to-date to avoid duplication.

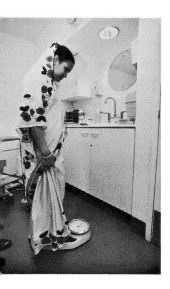

In the same way, your doctor can decide to take you off his or her list without giving a reason, although this is very uncommon, and will most probably be preceded by some kind of dispute or disagreement between you. If this happens, you can choose a new GP, or the FHSA will find one for you.

Having registered with a new GP, you should be offered a medical to check your weight, height and blood pressure. The doctor or nurse will also test your urine and ask a few questions about your family history and general health. This helps to get a picture of your health needs, and allows the doctor to suggest the best clinics for you to attend.

Getting the most from your GP

Being able to communicate well with your doctor is very important. You may find your doctor uses complicated language or does not bother to try to explain much to you. The pressure of time may make it impossible for you to describe fully what is wrong, or for your doctor to explain the recommended treatment and answer all your questions. Medical training is changing and putting more emphasis on the communication role of doctors. In the mean time, there are plenty of doctors who do not find this easy or just don't see it as important. Communication is a two-way process, and there are a number of things you can do to get the most from a visit to the GP.

Go well prepared with details of what is wrong, things that are worrying you, and questions you would like answered. Keep a note of when symptoms appear, what you have done about them, and whether anything has helped, and take this with you. Otherwise, everything may go completely out of your head when you are there. If you like, rehearse what you are going to say. Don't forget to mention any treatments or drugs you are receiving from elsewhere, and any other relevant information. You will also need to answer your doctor's questions as accurately as you can, even if they seem irrelevant.

Try not to feel pressured to get through the consultation too quickly. Doctors are busy, but time spent sorting something out early on can save time later. While the average consultation lasts about four minutes, this should be flexible.

If you don't understand what your doctor is saying, ask her to explain it again, and question anything you are not clear about. Vital information may be given when we are not in a position to understand it fully or remember it. Taking a few notes of the main points may help you think through what has been said once you get home. Hang on to these notes – you may want to refer to them again.

It may help to take someone with you for support when you visit your doctor. Choose someone you trust well enough to share confidential health information with, and who will help you say what you want to say and get answers to your questions. We are at our most vulnerable when we are ill and having someone there to argue our case if necessary can be helpful.

'I'd been very anxious about going back to my GP for the results of the biopsy. I knew things were serious, and that I might be in for bad news. I asked my sister to go with me – she was the only one who knew I was having tests, and was a great support. In the event, it was good news. We went for a drink after to celebrate. But I know I couldn't have faced the doctor on my own.'

If you are given a prescription, check that you know how and when to take it, how long for, and any reactions you may experience (see Medicines and prescriptions, pages 305-307).

Once a diagnosis has been made, possibly after test results are received, you should be given the chance to discuss treatment options. You need to be sure you understand the treatment and feel happy about the plan of action. If you need to be referred to a specialist, ask if there is a choice about where you go, and check that you know how long you may have to wait before you're seen.

If you feel you need to go away and think about what your doctor has said before making any decisions, tell her so and make an appointment for a return visit.

If you still feel unhappy about your doctor despite making all these efforts to help the relationship work, then you may need to consider finding an alternative practice, or seeking a second opinion (see below).

Sorting out problems with your GP

If you are dissatisfied with the advice your GP is offering, or with her attitude towards you, it's best to try to sort it out directly first. There may have been a misunderstanding or temporary break down in communication which can be put right. If you are unable to solve the problem this way, there are a number of steps you can take:

- Although you don't have an absolute right to a second opinion, your doctor will always be happy to refer you if she feels your request is reasonable.
- Make a formal complaint through the FHSA (Family Health Service Authority). If you want help with this, contact your Community Health Council.
- If you feel your doctor has behaved unethically or unprofessionally, for example, through neglect, incompetence, or a drink problem, you can complain to the General Medical Council (GMC), 44 Hallam Street, London W1.
- Decide to change GPs (see Choosing a GP practice, pages 297-299).

Other members of the primary health care team

Primary health care, so-called because it is to do with keeping us well and preventing illness, may be provided by a team of health professionals working together, and the cornerstone of that team is the GP. Other members of the primary care team include health visitors, community nurses, practice nurses, surgery or health centre receptionists, midwives, social workers, physiotherapists, and others. The team may be housed together under one roof, as is often the case in health centres. Or the GP practice may liaise with other health workers and refer you on to whoever you need to see. Most primary health care workers can also be contacted directly if you wish. Many different professionals may be included in the primary health care team, but some of the ones you are more likely to come across are described here.

- Practice nurses are employed by GPs to provide services such as taking blood samples, cervical smears, or providing family planning advice within the practice. They may also run support groups or clinics on topics such as premenstrual syndrome, menopause, weight control or smoking cessation.
- Health visitors work mainly with babies and children under 5, and with elderly people.
- Midwives take care of women during a normal pregnancy, birth, and for ten days after. You will see a midwife during your antenatal care, either at the GP practice or in hospital. If you decide to have a home delivery, a midwife will be allocated to you.
- Community nurses (or district nurses) provide practical nursing services in your home, for example, helping with bathing, changing dressings, giving injections.
- Chiropodists provide foot care, and will do home visits if the patient is housebound. Your GP will refer you for treatment, unless you are over 60, under 16, pregnant or have a disability, when you can go direct.
- Community psychiatric nurses provide support, information and nursing care to people with mental illness at home, and help with the transition of patients from hospital to home.

GP services

GP practices vary widely in the services they offer. A single-handed practice may provide little more than consultations with a doctor for diagnosis and minor treatment, or referral on to others. At the other end of the spectrum, the GP may work as a member of a team of professionals offering a variety of skills and services. The following services may be available at your GP practice:

- Contraceptive services. Most GPs provide contraceptive services, and more than 70 per cent of women use them. The whole range of family planning methods may not be available. Few GPs provide condoms, and many are uncertain about prescribing emergency contraception, which can be used up to 72 hours after having sex. While both GPs and practice nurses may offer contraceptive advice and treatment, this does not guarantee that they have had specific training in family planning.

- Pregnancy testing. Not all GPs offer this service, since they do not get paid for it through the NHS.

- Smear testing. All women between the ages of 20 and 64 are offered a free cervical smear test. (See section on Cervical cancer, pages 173-178.)

- Health promotion clinics. Some practices offer health promotion clinics on a number of health topics, such as smoking, diabetes, or weight control. They are usually run by the practice nurse, and you may be seen on a one-to-one basis, or in a group with others with a similar problem.

- Well-Women clinics. A number of services such as contraceptive advice, smear testing, blood pressure checks, HRT treatment, breast screening and cholesterol testing may be offered by the GP or practice nurse (see Well-Women services, pages 307-308)

- Child health surveillance. If you have children under 5 your GP may provide child health surveillance at regular intervals. Doctors have been offered a financial incentive to achieve certain targets for preventive health care such as immunisation and vaccination.

- Patient participation groups. A few practices offer these as a way of inviting discussion with patients about practice arrangements, or about specific health care issues. You could always approach your GP to set one up if you feel it would be useful. Routine consultations. If you have joined a new GP practice, your doctor should interview you to obtain your medical history and give some health advice. All patients over 75 should receive a home visit at least once a year.

Medicines and prescriptions

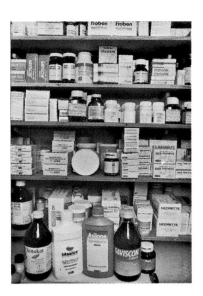

The pharmaceutical industry makes huge profits each year, and is at the heart of health-care services in the UK, promoting 'a pill for every ill'. In 1984, the NHS drugs bill was around £2,000 million, and it rises every year. With drug companies spending an enormous amount of time and money promoting their products to the medical profession, it is tempting for doctors to try one product after another to achieve a desired effect. The result is that we commonly find ourselves leaving the surgery with a prescription. If the first choice doesn't help, we will probably be offered a succession of others in what seems like rather a hit-and-miss approach. New drugs coming on to the market have to satisfy the Committee on the Safety of Medicines that they are safe and of a reasonable quality. But they do not have to show conclusively that they work better or as well as existing drugs. You may be asked to try out a new drug but your doctor has to ask for your written consent if this is part of a drug trial.

A particular treatment is more likely to work if you understand what is being offered, why it has been chosen, and what effect it may have. If you have a doctor who takes the time to discuss different options with you and explain what effects, good and bad, a particular drug may have, you are much more likely to stick to the instructions given and see a course of medication through. Many people, on the other hand, fail to take medication as directed or give up on it too quickly.

For minor ailments such as coughs, colds or period pains, we are increasingly encouraged to buy over-the-counter remedies – pharmacists are highly trained and usually willing to offer advice about the best medicine to choose. Be sure to give any relevant information, such as if you are pregnant, or taking a prescribed drug. Generic drugs – those that do not have brand names – work out much cheaper for the same effect, so look out for these.

If your doctor prescribes a medicine for you or someone you care for, there are a number of things that it is helpful to know:

- what is the medicine for, and what effect will it have?

- are there any side-effects to look out for, and what should you do if they occur?

- is there anything you should avoid while taking the medicine – certain foods, drinks – including alcohol, other medicines; driving or operating machinery, for example?

- how and when should you take it – with food, after food? What if you miss a dose?

- where should you store it, and what should you do with any left over?

- how long should you continue the treatment, and should you see the doctor again?

'My doctor told me I needed a tranquilliser to see me through a difficult patch. I wasn't too keen on the idea, but I desperately needed some kind of help. When I went back some weeks later, he offered a repeat prescription with hardly any questions about how I was doing. But I don't want to keep on taking pills if I don't need to.'

If you don't understand how you should take a drug, or why it has been prescribed, then don't be afraid to ask, and jot down notes if it will help you remember. It's annoying to get home and realise that you're not sure about whether to take it before or after a meal, at regular times or only when you have symptoms, and for how long. It's not unreasonable to phone the surgery to check up on any of these details – or check with your pharmacist. Where medicines are prescribed for your child, you may also want to find out:

- What types of preparations are available – soluble tablets, liquid suspensions, flavours, sugar-free options.

- Are there any alternative treatments, and why has this one been chosen?

- How will you know if the medicine is working? How long may this take? What warning signs should you look out for?

- When should you bring the child back to see the doctor again?

Where you or someone you care for needs to take a number of different medicines, things can get quite complicated. It may help to keep a record of all the medicines to be taken, when, and in what quantity. Your pharmacist will help you sort this out, and may help you to fill in a treatment plan.

Other Services in the Community

Well-Women services

You may be lucky enough to have a Well-Women service available locally. These vary in the type of services they offer, some having a fairly medical feel to them with a limited range of services, while others being run by and for women in a much more informal and flexible way. In many places they simply don't exist. If there's nothing where you live, you may find one close to where you work. To find out about them, look out for information in the local press, shops and libraries, surgeries and health centres, or ask the Community Health Council.

Well-Women services may be run by lay workers, often volunteers, and health professionals side-by-side. You will usually be offered the option of seeing a woman doctor if you wish. Most services offer cervical screening, pregnancy testing and contraceptive care. Some may also offer advice on topics such as breast self-examination, weight control and smoking cessation. Most are non-treatment oriented, referring you on to your GP, health centre, social services or other appropriate agency if need be.

Others have a much broader remit, providing health information on lots of different topics, drop-in sessions with crèche facilities, telephone help lines, discussion groups and self-help groups on anything from menopause and stress management to premenstrual syndrome, eating disorders and tranquillisers. Trained counsellors may be available to help with any health problem you want to bring them – bereavement, rape, abortion or even housing problems. There may be no professional input at all, with all work being carried out by lay workers and volunteers. Again, you will be referred on for any treatment needed. There may be a partnership between lay and professional workers, with one or more health workers available including doctors, health visitors, community psychiatric nurses or psychologists.

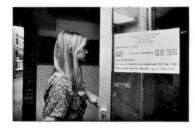

Unlike other health services, Well-Women services may try to make themselves as easy for you to get to and use as possible. Opening hours vary, but some offer evening and weekend sessions which are great if you work or have other daytime commitments. Many provide a crèche so that if you have young children you can still get the help you need without the interruptions and stress of taking them in with you. In some places, the service actually comes to you in the form of a mobile unit (usually a caravan or bus) which visits housing estates, shopping centres and workplaces.

Family planning clinics

With the current shortage of funds in the NHS, many family planning clinics have been closed over recent years. However, those still in existence offer a comprehensive range of contraceptive services, and many also provide pregnancy testing and cervical screening. The contraceptive advice and supplies are free. The doctors and nurses at these clinics will have had special training in family planning methods, and will be knowledgeable about the latest developments.

You can go along with your partner if you wish, and clinics tend to be more anonymous than a GP surgery. Some are walk-in, but for most you will need to make an appointment. To find your nearest family planning clinic, look in the phone book under 'family planning', or ask your GP, health centre, Community Health Council or FHSA (see Chapter Three).

Self-help groups

These are small informal groups of women who meet together to support each other and share experiences and information relevant to their health. Because they are run by women themselves rather than by a doctor or other health professional, they can approach a topic in any way they like, challenge or question medical practice, and explore a variety of options including alternative health care.

Some self-help groups are formed around specific health issues such as hysterectomy or ME (myalgic encephalomyelitis); others are more general, and give women the chance to talk about anything which they feel is relevant to their health, perhaps looking at common themes such as ways of being more assertive in personal relationships, or relationships with the medical profession and other authority figures. One particularly striking feature of self-help groups is that by sharing experiences women come to see how common their particular problem is, and feel less isolated. Strong friendships and support networks often develop out of such groups.

Health information centres

In some places, voluntary organisations arrange a service to provide women with easy access to health information. They may have a comprehensive library, and some provide telephone help lines. They are usually staffed by volunteers. Some also work for improvements in women's health services, campaign on women's health issues, and provide support to self-help groups.

Alternative Health Care

What are alternative therapies?

Alternative therapies are certainly not new! Many treatments and remedies have been developed and used in different parts of the world over many centuries. Most are based on a 'holistic' approach – viewing you as a whole person rather than treating just the one part that has gone wrong. The main ideas which underpin the different therapies are: the body has the capacity to heal itself, given the right support; it is finely balanced and illness occurs when it gets out of balance; and the way we live affects our health, so that changing our lifestyle may prevent illnesses recurring.

Alternative therapies are also often referred to as complementary therapies because they are seen to complement rather than to replace the range of traditional treatments on offer, so providing us with more options. Rather than bringing speedy cures, alternative therapies often need time, and may work best if combined with other approaches such as relaxation or a particular diet. By focusing on prevention and identifying the root cause of problems, they can help prevent the same condition occurring again and again. And they are cheaper to provide than conventional medicine which relies so heavily on expensive drugs and surgery.

Alternatives on the increase

Many women are not satisfied with the deal they get from the medical profession, and are looking elsewhere for help with staying healthy, treatment for certain conditions and relief from many others for which there is no cure. Fortunately we no longer have to rely only on orthodox treatments. Alternative therapies are much more widely available. A great number of people today have either consulted an alternative practitioner themselves or know someone who has. A recent survey in the UK showed most of us would be prepared to try a natural remedy, and more than half believe alternative therapies are effective.

Alternative therapies seem to have a particular appeal to women – we make up around two-thirds of the people who consult a natural practitioner. Maybe their appeal lies in the fact that alternative therapies see us as a whole person rather than trying to compartmentalise and medicalise the various biological events which are a natural part of life for many of us – periods, pregnancy, childbirth and the menopause. And we also especially welcome the way alternative therapies involve us as partners in our health care, so that we have a more equal relationship with the therapist and feel less powerless.

'I was tired of going to my doctor and not being listened to. I felt that without the insight and information I had to offer about my illness, he was just stabbing in the dark with different drugs and advice. The homeopathist I saw was so different – she spent a lot of time finding out about not just my symptoms but also about me as a person and events in my life. I felt like we were working together to get to the bottom of the problem.'

The medical profession is also beginning to take a more serious look at alternative therapies. Alongside their growing popularity with the public, some therapies are gaining in credibility with doctors as they realise that orthodox medicine does not have all the answers. Recent studies show that an increasing number of doctors feel the medical training they receive has limitations, and a growing number accept that alternative therapies have a contribution to make. While some feel that treatments should be carried out by doctors, others now accept the role of qualified lay practitioners, and are prepared to refer their patients to them.

The British Medical Association (BMA) is a professional organisation representing all doctors in the UK, and part of their role is to safeguard the public against possible harm to their health. In 1986 they published a fairly damning report on alternative therapies, dismissing them as ineffective and potentially harmful. Things have moved on since then and a new report, 'Complementary medicine – new approaches to good practice', published by the BMA in 1993, has taken a much less critical view, recommending the need for more research, a single regulating body for each therapy, and closer collaboration between doctors and alternative therapists in the treatment of patients.

Going for alternative therapies

You may be fed up with your doctor not listening to you, disenchanted with the high-tech approach of modern medicine, or yearning for more natural remedies which treat you as a whole person. If any or all of these are the case, you may be considering alternative therapies. Clearly, they are not right for everyone or for every illness, but they have much to offer that conventional medicine does not. And you don't have to think of it as an either/or situation – you may choose to use alternative therapies alongside more conventional treatment, to help relieve symptoms or cope better with them.

Orthodox medicine may be what is needed in your particular case. If you have new symptoms which have not been diagnosed, it's probably sensible to go first to your GP to find out whether you have any serious condition which requires medical treatment. You can then decide whether to opt for alternative treatment either on its own or as a complement to other treatment.

For everyday debilitating complaints like thrush, cystitis and menstrual problems, conventional treatments are far from adequate, and alternative therapies can offer an effective first line of treatment – and may be better at preventing the problem from coming back again and again. If you have a problem which recurs frequently – like PMS, migraine, or difficulty sleeping – you may be concerned about the effects of taking the medications, which orthodox treatments rely on, over a long period of time, possibly years, or about the possibility of different medicines you take reacting badly together. Alternative therapies, on the other hand, may be less likely to harm you, even when used over a long time - and they also may be better at getting to the cause of the problem so that it goes away.

'I'd been going to my doctor with cystitis on and off over the last four years. She always prescribed a course of antibiotics which usually knocked the cystitis on the head but left me with severe attacks of thrush. The homeopath I went to gave me treatment in the form of pills and a cream for external use, and it got rid of the cystitis without leaving me with thrush.'

Some illnesses continue to baffle doctors and treatment is sometimes far from ideal – it may have unpleasant or harmful side-effects, or may be unreliable in bringing about a cure. Some health problems such as ME , AIDS, certain types of cancer and many allergy-related complaints do not yet have effective orthodox treatments. It's true that alternative therapies can't work miracles either, but they offer a gentler approach and with far fewer known adverse effects. They may offer help and relief from some more unpleasant symptoms even if they cannot provide an absolute cure. And they can provide a useful back-up for stressful orthodox treatments such as surgery, radiotherapy or chemotherapy, helping your body to deal with the problem itself, and helping you cope with any unpleasant side-effects.

For some women, conventional treatments may be unsuccessful, leaving them to turn to alternative therapies as a last resort. If all else has failed, you may feel it worth while giving a different approach a try. Whether your problem is life-threatening, debilitating or merely a nuisance, there is little to lose from considering an alternative approach. Even if treatments offer no promise of a cure, they may well be able to improve your quality of life, helping you cope and making you feel more in control.

If you are considering alternative therapies, you may like to think about:

- what orthodox treatment options you have been offered
- what you have tried so far, and whether it helped
- whether there have been any unpleasant or worrying side-effects
- if you are confident about what your doctor is offering, or are you

worried about some aspect of the treatment offered

- if there are any alternative therapies that others have found useful for your complaint
- how you feel about trying something new
- if you want to be more involved in your treatment, and are thinking about changing aspects of your lifestyle.

Are alternative therapies safe and effective?

The main question you may be asking yourself when considering whether to try an alternative therapy is whether it is safe. In the UK, anyone can offer alternative therapies, whether or not they have undergone any form of training, as long as they don't make out that they are a registered medical practitioner. There are no comprehensive professional bodies to ensure standards are maintained and with whom you can lodge complaints. So how can you protect yourself from incompetent or unskilled therapists who may harm or injure you, use an inappropriate therapy for your condition, or result in you delaying seeking necessary orthodox treatments? The main things to remember are:

- see your GP with any new symptoms to check that you don't need any orthodox treatment, and to let them know what therapy you are planning to use
- choose a therapist carefully (see 'Finding a therapist, pages 318-320)
- if your problem doesn't clear up, go back to your doctor for help, or seek the advice of another therapist.

You will also be interested in whether the treatment you opt for is likely to be effective – especially as you will probably be paying for it. More studies are being carried out to find out about alternative therapies, how effective they are and any dangers which they may pose. Because of the way in which alternative therapies work, orthodox medical trials are not always appropriate, and new ways to evaluate them are needed. But some encouraging results are coming out of studies to date. For example, in 1990, research into patients with back pain found that those receiving chiropractic treatment improved by 70 per cent more than those given conventional treatment at a hospital outpatient department. Acupuncture has been found to be effective in relieving pain in 60 per cent of people suffering from chronic pain. And trials using homeopathy in the treatment of cystitis and rheumatoid arthritis have shown beneficial results.

Different therapies explained

Just what are all the different therapies and which one may be best for your condition? The following provides information about some of the more commonly used therapies to help you decide for yourself. There is not the space here to provide information on the many others available. To find out about which treatments are useful for which conditions, about professional bodies and who is qualified to carry out such treatments, you can contact the addresses for complementary and alternative medical practice at the end of this book.

Acupuncture

Background • This was developed by the Chinese, and is based on the idea that health is maintained by a balance of positive and negative energy in the body. It aims to treat the cause of symptoms by considering you as a whole person.

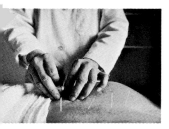

Treatment • Tiny needles are inserted into various parts of the body to stimulate points on 'energy lines', called meridians, each of which affects different organs. The needles may be left there for anything from a few seconds to an hour. This helps restore a balance, so relieving symptoms and stimulating energy forces. Before treatment, you will be asked about your medical history, lifestyle and emotional health. A physical examination will help to identify appropriate points to place the needles.

Useful for	•	A wide range of acute and chronic conditions. Particularly useful for relieving pain, for example, for headaches, period pains and endometriosis. It can also be used during childbirth and for stress-related problems such as depression.
What will it cost?	•	A first visit may cost about £30; subsequent visits will cost less.

Aromatherapy

Background	•	First developed by the ancient Egyptians, and later developed in France. One of the fastest-growing alternative therapies in recent years, used mainly by women.
Treatment	•	Essential oils are extracted from different parts of plants, and diluted before use either as cold compresses, for inhalation, in baths, or most often in massage. You will be asked about your health and how you feel. The therapist will select which essential oils to use, mix them with a few drops of vegetable oil, and use them to massage you.
Useful for	•	A wide variety of conditions for both mind and body. Especially effective for any stress-related complaints, period problems, problems connected with the menopause, and arthritis.
What will it cost?	•	Around £15-£30 per hour for a full body massage.

Herbalism

Background	•	Plants and plant extracts have been used to prevent and treat illness throughout history. They are also the basis of many modern medicines.
Treatment	•	Different parts of the plant may be used, including leaves, stems, seeds, flowers and roots, and preparations include tablets, teas and ointments. Your first consultation with a herbalist will involve an in-depth discussion

of your medical and personal history before herbal medicines are prescribed. If you are taking any other medicines or have a serious health problem, check with a qualified medical herbalist, your GP or pharmacist. Use over-the-counter herbal remedies to treat yourself only for very minor conditions. Products with the letters 'PL' (product licence) have been passed for safety and quality by the Department of Health.

Useful for
- A wide range of conditions, for example, painful, heavy or irregular periods; PMS; migraine; vaginal infections; menopausal problems such as hot flushes, night sweats and vaginal dryness; cystitis; and, in some cases, infertility can be treated. Also, acne, asthma, colds, burns and nervous complaints.

What will it cost?
- A first visit may cost around £20, and following visits will cost less.

Homeopathy

Background
- Based on the idea of treating like with like. Illnesses are treated with the very substances that cause the symptoms. The more dilute the substance, the more potent it is. This mobilises the body's own defences to fight the cause of the problem.

Treatment
- You will be asked about your moods and emotions, likes and dislikes, before being given a remedy specific for you. Available from doctors who have homeopathic training, or professional homeopaths with no formal medical training but who have completed an approved four-year course. Your GP could refer you as an NHS patient to one of five homeopathic hospitals (in Bristol, Glasgow, Liverpool, London and Tunbridge Wells). Over-the-counter homeopathic remedies are all right for minor complaints and first aid. Never attempt to treat a serious condition with shop-bought remedies.

Useful for
- Most illnesses, including bladder infections, cysts and fibroids, menstrual

problems, headaches, stress, anxiety and depression.

What will it cost? • A first visit may cost between £20 and £50. Subsequent visits will be less. You may be able to get homeopathic treatment free on the NHS.

Osteopathy and chiropractic

Background • Both have ancient origins, practised by the Greeks, Romans and others. They involve manipulating and adjusting the spine and other joints. If the spine is not in proper alignment it interferes with the nerve and blood flow to other areas, causing disease.

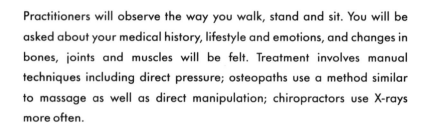

Treatment • Practitioners will observe the way you walk, stand and sit. You will be asked about your medical history, lifestyle and emotions, and changes in bones, joints and muscles will be felt. Treatment involves manual techniques including direct pressure; osteopaths use a method similar to massage as well as direct manipulation; chiropractors use X-rays more often.

Useful for • Back and neck weaknesses, spinal and joint disorders, headaches. Chiropractic may also help with menstrual problems, insomnia, sciatica, lumbago, constipation and bladder problems.

What will it cost? • A first visit to an osteopath will cost around £20 to £30, with following hourly sessions from £12 to £30. Chiropractic treatment costs from £12 to £20, and X-rays can cost an extra £30.

Finding a therapist

Very few alternative therapies are available on the NHS. But, as treatments gain respect from the medical establishment, the situation is improving. It's worth asking your GP what's available in your area. Since April 1992 GP's have been free to employ alternative practitioners in their practices, so some treatments may even be available at your surgery or health centre. If your own GP is not very helpful, your FHSA (Family Health Service Authority) will be able to tell you of other GP practices in your area offering alternative therapy.

'My GP Practice offers homeopathy and acupuncture within the practice. I was very surprised when he suggested acupuncture to treat my endometriosis. I was a little sceptical at first, but was in such a lot of pain that I would have tried anything. The results have been dramatic.'

It's sometimes difficult to find out exactly what different treatments there are, and which ones may be best for your condition. (You could contact the Institute of Complementary Medicine, see Useful organisations, at the end of this book). An increasing number of alternative health centres, and even some orthodox ones, offer a number of different therapies under one roof. You will probably see an orthodox doctor first, and together decide which therapy or combination of therapies will suit your particular needs. This mixing and matching of therapies may be particularly useful for some conditions where a number of different approaches are needed.

For most therapies you will have to pay, although many practitioners offer a sliding scale of fees, so that you pay in relation to what you can afford. Choosing a therapist can be difficult – how do you know if they are any good? And how much will your treatment cost? No central register or directory of practitioners exists, and practitioners are not obliged to belong to any organisation. But efforts are now being made to standardise training, and to ensure any remedies and treatments offered are safe and effective. And while anyone can set up as a therapist, in practice training standards are high and improving all the time.

You need to find someone who is competent, has the necessary training, and won't cost the earth. Your doctor may be able to recommend a therapist, or personal recommendation from a friend is a good way of choosing someone – if you feel confident about what they can offer you're halfway there. Alternatively, you can contact one of the national organisations (listed under the different therapies at the end of this book) for names of practitioners in your area, or look in your local phone book or newspapers for practitioners advertising their services. It may be helpful to consider the following points:

Think about:
- will this therapy be useful for my condition?
- is the therapist registered?
- what about his/her training and qualifications?
- does he/she come recommended?
- how much will be charged per session, and how long is the treatment likely to take?

Using self-help remedies

Alternative therapies offer a range of treatments which you can use to help yourself for minor ailments and injuries. Anything more serious needs the attention of a qualified practitioner. Any condition that does not clear up quickly should be referred to a doctor or therapist.

Herbal remedies can offer simple self-help treatments for many minor ailments. If you are taking any other medicines, the herbal treatment may affect the way they work.

Aromatherapy is also an easy treatment to use for yourself at home, though be careful to avoid certain essential oils which can be harmful – including origanum, sage, thyme, savory and wintergreen. Certain others should not be used when you are pregnant – as well as those mentioned above, avoid black pepper, basil, clove, hyssop, marjoram, myrrh, camphor, cedarwood, juniper and pennyroyal.

There are a number of different homeopathic self-help remedies, but as with herbalism, you should only treat the most simple ailments yourself.

Private Heath Care

Weighing up the benefits

Private medical care is available either on a self-pay basis, or through health insurance, which you may buy yourself or may be provided as a perk by your employer.

Despite the high costs involved, many people are opting for private health care because they believe they will get faster, and in some cases superior, treatment. While most acute and emergency care is well provided for through the NHS, for less life-threatening conditions you may have to wait some time for NHS treatment. And there is growing concern that shortage of funds in the health service is leading to delays in more urgent treatments such as heart by-pass surgery, and biopsies to detect cancer.

Speed of treatment needs to be weighed against other factors. Many up-to-date treatments are available only in teaching and research hospitals within the NHS, whereas private medical care is often provided in privately run clinics and hospitals. If you have private medical care and develop complications which cannot be dealt with where you are, you may need to be transferred to NHS facilities which can cope with your problem. For example, private maternity care may be fine for a trouble-free delivery, but if you or your baby need emergency medical treatment you may have to be moved quickly to another hospital, with all the risks and trauma which that involves.

In order to get private medical care, you need to be referred by a GP in the same way as if you were using the NHS. Going private certainly has a number of advantages:

- a quicker initial appointment with a consultant, especially important if you are in pain or worried about symptoms.

- treatment, including surgery, if necessary, at a time to suit you, which is helpful if you have work, family or social commitments which you need to work round.

- comfortable surroundings, including a room on your own or with a few others, food menus, free visiting and pleasant facilities.

Health insurance

What it covers

Depending on the insurance cover which you take out, it may:

- meet the cost (or part of the cost, up to a pre-determined limit) of private medical treatments for which you are covered

- cover the cost of out-patient appointments, X-rays and tests

- make cash payments to those members who receive treatment in the NHS

- cover the cost of other treatments necessary for your recovery, such as physiotherapy, providing your consultant recommends it.

You are usually not covered for:

- GP appointments
- routine dental work
- normal pregnancy
- medical conditions which you were known to suffer from before taking out the insurance.

Choosing health insurance

Various companies offer health care insurance. The bigger ones like BUPA and PPP are widely known, but there are others too. It's important to read all the small print and understand how you can and cannot use the insurance, what is covers, and what the conditions of joining are.

The cost of different schemes varies widely, reflecting the different cover offered. For example, some schemes only cover the cost of medical care if you cannot receive the same treatment under the NHS within a certain time, usually about six weeks. Check what procedures (surgical or medical) are covered, and what is the financial limit.

Making a claim

Insurance policies will require you to complete a form, and there will also be a section for your GP and/or your consultant to complete. The form will request information about what is wrong with you, what your GP recommends, when you first consulted him or her for this particular problem, if you were referred by your GP, and what treatment or surgery is recommended.

Your Rights in the NHS

Traditionally we have not been very good at sticking up for our rights for health care. When the NHS was first introduced, people were grateful for whatever it had to offer. But more people today are aware of their rights and are demanding higher standards, expecting the health service to be just that – a service to meet their needs.

So what rights do you have? On 1 April 1992, the Patients' Charter came into being, and it sets out clearly your legal rights to care in the NHS. It states that we all have the right:

- to receive health care on the basis of clinical needs, regardless of our ability to pay
- to be registered with a GP
- to receive emergency medical care at any time (through a GP, or emergency ambulance service and hospital accident and emergency services)

- to be referred to a consultant (acceptable to you) when your GP thinks it necessary, and to be referred for a second opinion if you and your GP agree this is desirable

- to be given a clear explanation of any treatment proposed (including any risks and any alternatives) before you decide whether you will agree to the treatment

- to have access to your health records, and to know that those working for the NHS are under a legal duty to keep their contents confidential

- to choose whether or not you wish to take part in medical research or medical student training

- to be given detailed information of local health services, including quality standards and maximum waiting times – available from the District Health Authority, your GP, and your local Community Health Council

- to be guaranteed admission for treatment by a specific date no later than two years from the day when your consultant places you on a waiting list; this is the responsibility of the district Health Authority, and your GP

- to have any complaint about NHS services (whoever provides them) investigated, and to receive a full and prompt reply from the chief executive or general manager. If you remain unhappy about your complaint you have a right to take the matter up with the Health Service Commissioner.

In addition to our legal rights, some National Charter Standards have been identified for the NHS to achieve, as far as circumstances and resources allow. These include:

- respect for privacy, dignity and religious and cultural beliefs

- arrangements to ensure everyone (including people with special needs) can use NHS services

- information should be given to relatives and friends

- waiting times for an ambulance service should be no more than fourteen minutes in an urban area, and nineteen minutes in a rural area

- in an accident and emergency department, you should be seen immediately and your need for treatment assessed

- in an outpatient clinic, you should be seen within thirty minutes of a specific appointment time

- your operation should not be cancelled on the day you are due to arrive in hospital (except because of emergencies or staff sickness)

- a qualified nurse, midwife or health visitor should be responsible for each patient

- on discharge of patients from hospital, your hospital will agree arrangements for meeting decisions made regarding any continuing health or social care.

At a local level, health authorities also set and publicise local standards which they aim to meet, including waiting times for first outpatient appointments and in accident and emergency departments; the waiting time for taking you home after you have been treated (where your doctor says you have a medical need for NHS transport); making it easier for you and your visitors to find your way around hospitals, by providing enquiry points and better signposting; and ensuring staff you meet face-to-face wear name badges.

Making a complaint

If you are unhappy about services you have received, for example you had to wait two hours for an ambulance, or the result of a smear test was mislaid and you had to chase it up, you should write to: Duncon Nichol (Chief Executive of the NHS), Department of Health, Richmond House, 79 Whitehall, London SW1A 2NS

Health Care at Work

Women at work

Around 26 million people in the UK are in full-time employment, and nearly half of these workers are women. We spend a large proportion of our time at work, and the environment we work in and facilities available to us there can have an important impact on our health. Depending on the size of your firm, your health needs may be covered by a first-aid box at one end of the spectrum to a comprehensive medical service at the other. Your workplace may also have a number of policies affecting your health – for example, a no-smoking policy, no-alcohol policy, healthy eating policy, and policies relating to pregnancy, maternity leave and child care.

Under the 1974 Health and Safety at Work Act, employers have to ensure as far as possible a healthy and safe working environment for all employees. If you are covered by a recognised trade union, you have the right to elect safety representatives and a health and safety committee. If you suspect there are hazards where you work, you can call in an inspector from the Health and Safety Executive, or a local authority environmental health inspector, who will first try to *persuade* the employer to deal with any problems identified, or failing that to enforce the law.

Workplace screening initiatives

A growing number of employers are encouraging women employees to have breast and cervical cancer screening at regular intervals. A quarter of the UK's top firms now offer a screening facility. It's worth asking your personnel department or going through your union to find out what provisions there are for you. Ideally, you should be offered paid time off for screening regardless of age or length of service, and part-time staff should be included. There are two main options.

If you work for a small organisation or there are only a few women in your workplace, you may be able to get paid time off work to attend a local NHS screening centre, or you may be able to join with other women in a nearby workplace to use their screening facility.

If you are part of a large workforce with a significant number of female employees, it may be possible for a special mobile cancer screening unit to visit your workplace.

The Women's Nationwide Cancer Control Campaign have a fleet of mobile units and have visited 700 places of work in the last three years, screening 35,000 women.

You will be able to see a female doctor, and for some women the anonymity of the consultation makes it easier than going to their GP. In addition to a cervical smear test, you may be offered breast examination, instruction in breast awareness, an internal pelvic examination, and a blood pressure check. You will be given the result of the breast check at once, and results of the smear test will be sent directly to you, with a copy to your GP.

No-smoking policies

Your workplace may be one of the growing numbers to have a no-smoking policy. ASH (Action on Smoking and Health) estimates that one UK company in five has a formal written smoking policy, and up to 80 per cent of large firms have some sort of restrictions. Passive smoking has been found to be a cause of lung-cancer amongst non-smokers (see section on Passive smoking, pages 250-251). In Autumn 1992, the Health and Safety Executive published new guidance notes for employers, warning that passive smoking at work can damage non-smokers' health. It seems that the implications for workplace smoking may be profound, with employers no longer able to ignore the issue, and more and more developing comprehensive no-smoking policies.

In some workplaces, smoking is ruled out because of the nature of the job – food handling, or fire risks, for example. But in many, smoking is a different kind of problem. Employers are recognising the need to provide a smoke-free environment for the majority of their employees, and help for smokers who wish to give up.

Policies vary from one employer to another. They should be made clear to you when you are recruited, or if they are introduced at your existing place of work there should be a process whereby employees are consulted and fully informed. Your employer may choose to recruit only non-smokers, and to make the non-smoking policy part of your contract of employment. Breaches of the smoking policy may be made a matter for disciplinary procedure. Alternatively, policies may depend on voluntary agreements, which can lead to conflict between smoking and non-smoking staff. If you are concerned about other people's smoke where you work, you should seek help from your personnel department or union representative.

What the policy may cover

The policy may restrict smoking in the whole workplace, including offices, canteens, loos, lifts, stairways and workshops, for example, or it may only cover certain areas such as multi-occupancy rooms, meeting-rooms or public areas.

Special areas may be provided for use by smokers, and you may be allowed smoking breaks during work hours, although your employer is not obliged to provide them.

Smokers may be offered information about giving up smoking, or help with cessation through support groups, counselling, acupuncture or hypnotherapy. This may be provided in work time, or in your own time during a lunch break or after work. If you feel you need help of this kind and it hasn't been offered, ask for it. You could get together with other colleagues who smoke to request help, or offer each other support.

Alcohol policies

There is a growing recognition that drinking alcohol during working hours affects work performance and can cause health and safety risks. Sickness and absence from work related to drinking is estimated to cost industry around £800 million a year, and heavy drinkers take up to three times as many days off as other workers.

If you have recognised that you have a drink problem yourself, or know someone you work with has a problem, it may feel very risky to let someone else at work know – at worst you may fear losing your job or ruining your career prospects. Much depends on the attitude of your employer to alcohol – if there is a clear alcohol policy, the chances are that they have thought through the issues around problem drinking very carefully, and can offer some positive help and support for employees wishing to do something about their problem.

A number of workplaces are introducing alcohol policies, and some also offer education about sensible drinking and support for workers with a problem. A policy on drinking at work should apply to staff at every level, and clear information about the policy should be available, to include:

- support available for employees with a drink problem, and whether they may have time off on sick leave for recovery, with an opportunity to return to their job if possible.
- a policy regarding alcohol on the premises – for example, in the canteen or bar, social club or when entertaining at work.
- the role of managers in recognising and acting when they identify an employee as having a drink problem.

Repetitive strain injury

Anyone who does a job which involves repetitive movement is at risk.

Because of the large concentration of women in repetitive tasks, both in factories and offices, we are particularly at risk. Repetitive Strain Injury may cause discomfort or persistent pain in muscles, tendons and other soft tissues. Any work involving rapid repetitive movements, or awkward postures that are held for long periods of time, may cause RSI or make it worse.

Apart from your employer's general duties under the HSW Act to ensure the health and safety of employees, there are no specific legal requirements to prevent RSI. However, you can ask your employer for information, and get them to identify high risk tasks and redesign them to reduce risks.

Working with VDUs

Probably more than half the workforce in industrialised countries use visual display units (VDUs) on a regular basis. A large proportion of VDU workers are women, and there are concerns about the actual and possible health risks associated with VDUs.

VDU work can lead to a number of different health problems, including eye strain and RSI in fingers, hands, wrists or arms. At present, the link between VDUs and reproductive hazards is unproven. While more research is carried out, some countries allow pregnant women the right to move, if they choose, to other equivalent work not involving VDUs during their pregnancy, or to take leave during their pregnancy without loss of employment rights.

One of the best ways to reduce the risk encountered by VDU workers is to limit the time which an individual spends working on VDUs. An Economic Community Directive on Display Screen Equipment has introduced a range of measures, and the most significant of these mean that you should:

- interrupt your work on a display screen with regular breaks or changes of activity
- have an eye and eyesight test before starting work on display screens, and regularly thereafter
- receive information and training about VDU use
- have a working environment, display screen, keyboard, desk, chair, lighting and task design to minimise risk

If you are pregnant, or considering getting pregnant, and are concerned about the possible danger of working with VDUs, you should talk to your personnel officer or union representative about the possibility of transferring to other work, without the loss of pay, status, or career prospects.

Sexual and racial harassment

Both sexual and racial harassment can have profound effects on the lives of working women. Sexual harassment can include looks, jokes and comments, just as much as physical contact. Although it may be difficult to identify, it is any behaviour which you make clear is unwanted but which the harasser persists with. Remember that it is always your perception which is most important.

Racial harassment at work can take many forms. It can involve unfair decisions by your employer, repeated and unwelcome comments, and racist abuse through physical attack. Black women often experience both racial and sexual harassment, and for many black workers it can be an everyday occurrence in their working lives.

Harassment is a health and safety issue, because of the effect it may have on victims, making them feel isolated and stressed, perhaps leading to depression and physical illness and affecting their ability to do the job. It can also lead to absenteeism.

Find out what policy there is at your workplace, and what procedures there are for dealing with complaints. Ideally there should be an officer appointed to whom you can take problems of harassment, although this system sometimes does not work as it should. Your trade union representative should be able to help.

In Conclusion

This book has only been able to scratch the surface of women's health care issues. It does not cover specific issues like childbirth, to which many excellent books are already devoted. Nor does it comprehensively cover many of the health problems we share with men, or problems such as the everyday coughs and colds which make life miserable. It is not a comprehensive medical encyclopaedia but a guide which suggests an approach to your health and medical problems.

The approach to health and well-being in the preceding pages will allow you to get the most out of your body, whatever your age and whatever your circumstances.

To take control of your body is to take control of your life.

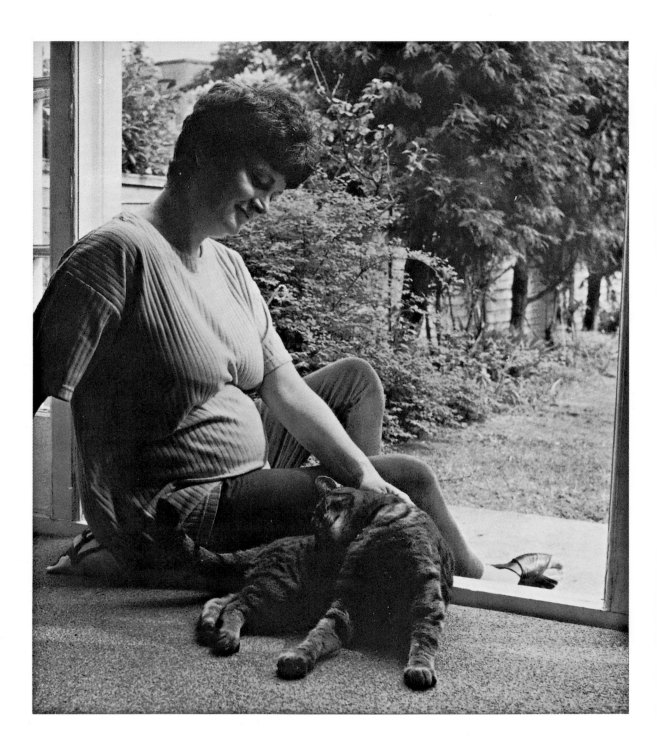

Abortion

British Pregnancy
Advisory Service
•   Austy Manor, Wootton Wawen, Solihull,
W Midlands B95 6BX
Telephone 0564 793225

Marie Stopes Clinics
•   108 Whitfield Street,
London W1P 6BE
Telephone 071 388 4843

Pregnancy Advisory
Service
•   11-13 Charlotte Street,
London W1P 1HD
Telephone 071 637 8962

Support After
Termination for
Abnormality (SATFA)
•   29/30 Soho Square,
London W1V 6JB
Telephone 071 439 6124

Alcohol and drug abuse

Al-Anon
•   61 Great Dover Street,
London SE1 4YF
Helpline 071 352 3001

Alcoholics Anonymous
•   Helpline 071 332 0202 (6-11 pm)

DAWN (Drugs and
Alcohol:
Women's Network)
•   c/o GLAAS, 30-31 Great Sutton Street,
London EC1V 0DX
Telephone 071 253 6221

Support After
Termination for
Abnormality (SATFA)
•   29/30 Soho Square,
London W1V 6JB
Telephone 071 439 6124

Bereavement

Cruse Bereavement Care • Cruse House, 126 Sheen Road, Richmond, Surrey TW9 1UR
Telephone 081 940 4818
Helpline: 081 332 7227 (Mon-Fri 9.30am-5 pm)

Cancer

Breast Cancer Care • Anchor House, Britten Street, London SW3 3TZ
Freephone helpline 0500 245345 Nationwide
Helpline 071 867 1103 London
Helpline 041 353 1050 Glasgow
Helpline 031 221 0407 Edinburgh

Breast Care and Mastectomy Association of Great Britain • 15-19 Britten Street, London SW3 3TZ
Helpline 071 867 1103
Freephone 0500 245345

Breast Care and Mastectomy Association of Great Britain (Scotland) • Suite 2/8, 65 Bath Street, Glasgow G2 2BX
Telephone 041 353 1050

British Association of Cancer United Patients (BACUP) • No. 3 Bath Place, Rivington Street, London EC2A 3JR
Telephone 071 696 9003
Counselling 071 608 1038
Freephone 0800 181 199

CancerLink • 17 Britannia Street, London WC1X 9JN
Telephone 071 833 2451/031 228 5557

The Skincare Campaign • 4 Tavistock Place, London WC1H 9RA
Telephone 071 713 0377

| The Women's Nationwide Cancer Control Campaign | • | Suna House, 128-130 Curtain Road, London EC2A 3AR Telephone 071 729 4688 |

Complementary and Alternative Medicine

| Aromatherapy Organisations Council | • | 3 Latymer Close, Braybooke, Market Harborough, Leicestershire LE16 8LN Telephone 0858 434242 |

| British Homeopathic Association | • | 27a Devonshire Street, London W1N 1RJ Telephone 071 935 2163 |

| Chiropractic Association | • | 29 Whitley Street, Reading RG2 0EG Telephone 0734 757557 |

| Council for Acupuncture | • | 179 Gloucester Place, London NW1 6DX Telephone 071 724 5756 |

| Council for Complementary and Alternative Medicine | • | 179 Gloucester Place, London NW1 6DX Telephone 071 724 9103 |

| General Council and Register of Osteopaths | • | 56 London Street, Reading RG1 4SQ Telephone 0734 576585 |

| The Institute for Complementary Medicine | • | PO BOX 194, London SE16 1QZ Telephone 071 237 5165 |

| International Federation of Aromatherapists | • | Royal Masonic Hospital, Ravenscourt Park, London W6 0TN Telephone 081 846 8066 |

National Institute of Medical Herbalists	• 9 Palace Gate, Exeter EX1 1JA Telephone 0392 426022
Society of Homeopaths	• 2 Artizan Road, Northampton NN1 4HU Telephone 0604 21400

Contraception

Brook Advisory Centres	• 153a East Street, London SE17 2SD Telephone 071 708 1234
Family Planning Association	• 27-35 Mortimer Street, London W1N 7RJ Helpline 071 636 7866 (Mon-Fri 10am to 3pm)

Coronary Heart Disease

Coronary Prevention Group	• Plantation House, 31-35 Fenchurch Street, London EC3M 3NN Telephone 071 626 4844

Eating Disorders

The Eating Disorders Association	• Sackville Place, 44-48 Magdalen Street, Norwich, Norfolk NR3 1JE (Send a stamped envelope)

Endometriosis

Endometriosis Society	• 35 Belgrave Square, London SW1X 8QB Telephone 071 235 4137

HIV/Aids

National Aids Helpline	• Telephone 0800 567 123 (Freephone 24 hours a day 7 days a week)

Terence Higgins Trust • Helpline 071 242 1010 (12 noon to 10 pm)

Infertility

Issue (formerly National Association for the Childless) • 509 Aldridge Road, Great Barr, Birmingham B44 8NA
Telephone 021 344 4414

Menopause

Hysterectomy Support Network • 3 Lynne Close, Green Street, Orpington, Kent BR6 6BS

Menopause Society • 83 High Street, Marlow,
Buckinghamshire SL7 1AB
Telephone 0628 890199

National Osteoporosis Society • PO Box 10, Radstock, Bath BA3 3YB
Telephone 0761 432 472

Miscarriage

The Miscarriage Association • Clayton Hospital, Northgate, Wakefield,
West Yorkshire WF1 3JS
(Send a stamped envelope)

Pregnancy

Maternity Alliance • 15 Britannia Street,
London WC1X 9JP
Telephone 071 837 1265

Premenstrual Syndrome

National Association for Premenstrual Syndrome

- PO Box 72, Sevenoaks, Kent TN13 3PS
  (Send a stamped envelope)

The Premenstrual Society

- PO Box 102, London SE1 7ES
  (Send a stamped envelope)

Sex and Relationships

Association of Sexual and Marital Therapists

- c/o Dr C. M. Duddle, Student Health Centre, University of Manchester, Manchester M13 9QS
  (Send a stamped envelope and the Association will forward the details of your nearest sex therapist or clinic)

British Association of Counselling

- 1 Regent Place, Rugby, Warwickshire CV21 2PJ
  Telephone 0788 578 328

Rape Crisis Centres Helpline

- Telephone 071 837 1600

Relate (formerly National Marriage Guidance)

- Herbert Gray College, Little Church Street, Rugby CV21 3AP
  Telephone 0788 573241

Support group for vaginismus sufferers

- Resolve, PO Box 820, London N10 3AW
  (Send a stamped envelope)

SPOD (Association to Aid the Sexual and Personal Relationships of People with a Disability)

- 286 Camden Road, London N7 OBJ.
  Telephone 071 607 8851

Smoking

ASH (Action on Smoking and Health)
- 109 Gloucester Place, London W1H 3PH
  Telephone 071 935 3519

Quit
- Victory House, 170 Tottenham Court Road, London W1P 0HA
  Telephone 071 388 5775
  Quitline 071 487 3000

Toxic Shock Syndrome

Women's Health
- 52 Featherstone Street, London EC1Y 8RT
  Telephone 071 251 6580

Women's Environmental Network
- Aberdeen Studios, 22 Highbury Grove, London N5 2EA
  Telephone 071 354 8823

Workplace

Repetitive Strain Injury Association
- Chapel House, 152-156 High Street, Yiewsley, West Drayton, Middlesex UB7 7BE
  Telephone 0895 431134

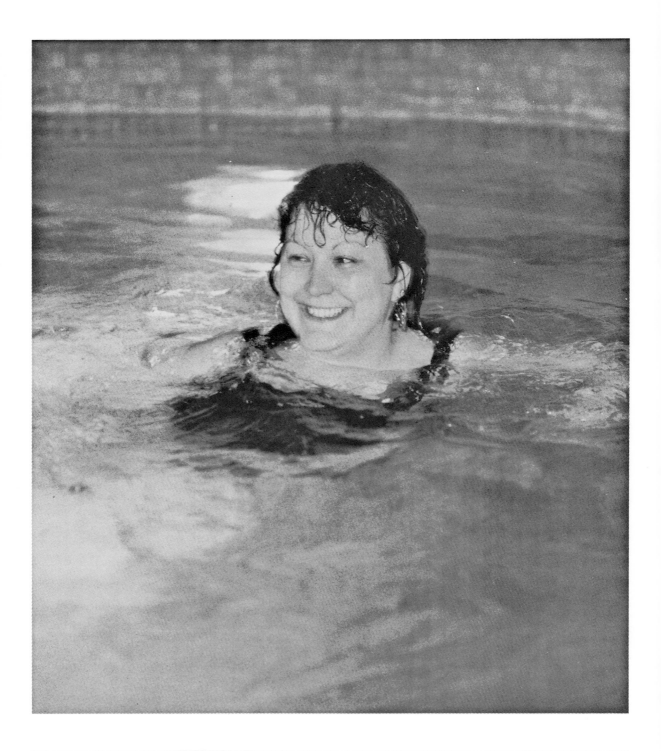

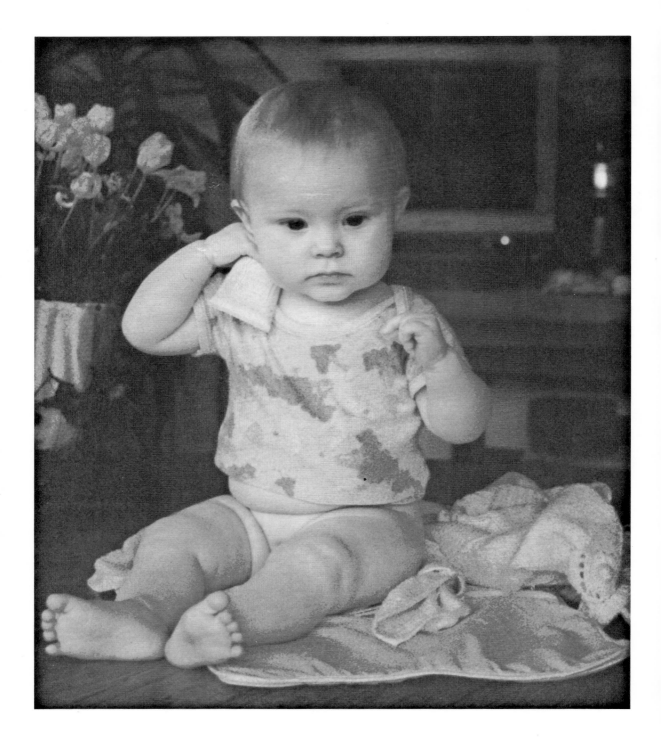

Locations

BSO (British School of Osteopathy)
1-4 Suffolk Street, London SW1

Britannia Leisure Centre
40 Hyde Road, London N1

Crowndale Health Centre
59 Crowndale Road, Camden, London NW1

Margaret Pyke Centre
15 Bateman Buildings, Soho Square, London W1

Maternity Unit (UCLH)
University College London Hospital, Huntley Street, London WC1

Women and Health
4 Carol St, Camden, London NW1

Models

Angela High
Polly High
Sue Johnston
Eldorna Mapp
Rosie Ruddock
Lucy Shipton

Agency Photographs

Sally & Richard Greenhill (pages 214, 286, 290)
Polly High (page 9)
Eileen Langsley (page 208)